THE RETURN OF DESIRE

OTHER BOOKS BY GINA OGDEN

The Heart and Soul of Sex
Women Who Love Sex
Food for Body and Soul
Sexual Recovery
Safe Encounters (coauthor)
When a Family Needs Therapy (coauthor)

The RETURN of DESIRE

A Guide to Rediscovering Your Sexual Passion

GINA OGDEN, PhD

TRUMPETER

BOSTON · 2008

To Isis
Supreme Lover
Initiator into the Sexual Mysteries
Restorer of Body and Soul

This book is intended as an educational volume only, not as a medical manual. The information given here is designed to help you make informed decisions about your health and pleasure. It is not intended as a substitute for any treatment that may have been prescribed by your doctor. If you suspect that you have a medical problem or if you experience emotional discomfort, we urge you to seek competent medical help or counseling from a skilled sexuality educator or therapist.

Trumpeter Books
An imprint of Shambhala Publications, Inc.
Horticultural Hall
300 Massachusetts Avenue
Boston, Massachusetts 02115
www.shambhala.com

© 2008 by Gina Ogden

Selection from the Goddess Chant, copyright © Shawna Carol. Reprinted by permission of Pagan People's Music.

A portion of the author's proceeds will be donated to organizations promoting women's health.

9 8 7 6 5 4 3 2 1

FIRST EDITION

Printed in the United States of America

♾ This edition is printed on acid-free paper that meets the American National Standards Institute z39.48 Standard.

Distributed in the United States by Random House, Inc., and in Canada by Random House of Canada Ltd

Library of Congress Cataloging-in-Publication Data

Ogden, Gina.
The return of desire: a guide to rediscovering your sexual passion / Gina Ogden.—1st ed.
p.   cm.
Includes bibliographical references and index.
ISBN 978-1-59030-364-1 (pbk.: alk. paper)
1. Sex instruction for women. 2. Women—Sexual behavior. 3. Sexual desire disorders. 4. Intimacy (Psychology) 5. Couples. I. Title.
HQ46.O43 2008
306.7082—dc22
2007045038

CONTENTS

INTRODUCTION

Refocusing the Conversation about Desire

THIS BOOK IS BASED ON what I've learned in over three decades as a sex therapist, educator, and researcher. It's also based on the 3,810 responses to the national survey I conducted on sexuality and spirituality, which explored a range of questions other sex surveys have not investigated. Instead of querying "how much," "how many," and "how often," I asked respondents how their sexual relationships felt to them and what they meant in their lives. My earlier book *The Heart and Soul of Sex* discusses the survey results—which indicate that sexual experience includes much more than we've been led to believe by doctors, religious leaders, media reporters, and Miss Morrison, when she caught us fiddling with ourselves in third grade. ("Class! We will now all place our hands on the tops of our desks—in full sight please!)

The Return of Desire continues where *The Heart and Soul of Sex* leaves off. It investigates sexual desire through the lens of relationship. The focus is on women—who we are, how we feel, and how our views of sex evolve as we mature, change our shape, our hair color, and perhaps our partners and our sexual lifestyles. It isn't that men's opinions don't count. It's that most models of sexual desire begin with men and end with women not quite measuring up. It's the old Mars-Venus view of the universe, where men are supposed to be the fixed sexual stars. So to focus on women, on what we feel and on what we can do to reclaim desire on our own terms, opens up a sexual cosmos that has never been fully explored.

Part 1 explores the many faces of sexual desire. It invites you to understand the richness and complexity of what women want—beyond performance, beyond hormones, beyond the medical model that polarizes function and dysfunction, and beyond the cultural clichés that polarize men and women. Here, you'll learn about the four energies that spark sexual desire, and how these relate to your relationships, including the all-important relationship you develop with yourself.

Part 2 investigates the myriad reasons women say no to sex. It leads you through some major passages and pitfalls of sexual desire—from falling in love, to affairs, pleasure anxiety, codependency, abuse, and "good old-fashioned Catholic guilt" (as one woman puts it). It addresses some specific problems women associate with sexual desire: Is it childbirth? Is it low self-worth? Is it men? Is it sexual orientation? Chapters in part 2 offer a breadcrumb path through all of these issues, with scores of practical ways to help you find your way home.

Part 3 suggests how you can expand your beliefs about sexual desire. It leads you to explore the notion of sacred union—the spiritual mysteries of sexual connection and meaning. This is a controversial path for many of us because we've been so accustomed to think of sexuality as separate from spirituality. Yet you'll hear from women—and men—who assert that sexual desire is a path to the divine, and vice versa—that opening up spiritually can awaken the deepest longings of the body. The afterword encourages you to create a new story—your own story—about sexual desire and all that it may mean for your life.

This book is a call to refocus the conversation about desire—onto the kinds of sexual relationships women really want. Throughout, I call on the wisdom of thousands of women of varying ages and lifestyles who have shared with me how they've discovered erotic pleasure in their relationships. I invite you to take their stories into your heart and use them as a blueprint for returning sexual desire to its rightful owner—you. And I invite you to pass your knowledge on to your intimate partner, or partners. If you are your own intimate partner, you can just smile inscrutably and keep this knowledge all for yourself.

Ultimately, *The Return of Desire* conveys the idea that our sexual relationships are multidimensional, life-giving, and transformative and that the most enduring qualities of sexual desire cannot be counted and measured. There's no one right formula for bringing the fullness of sexual desire into your life at any age. Nor is there one right standard for judging you as sexually deficient or dysfunctional if you don't feel hot for certain kinds of sexual activity—or for any sexual activity at all. You'll find information here to help you honor your own experience, and encourage you to appreciate all that you see in the mirror of your body, mind, heart, and soul.

You'll also find encouragement to step through the looking glass to a larger vision of sexual consciousness. Desire can mean more than just a good time on Saturday night. Nothing wrong with that of course. But desire can also be an ongoing wellspring of sensation, of connection, of hope. Desire can plunge us profoundly into ourselves and launch us galaxies beyond ourselves. Desire can lead us to understand that our most intimate relationships form a template for all our relationships—with community, with the environment, and with the realm of spirit. Too often we've denounced sexual desire as the proverbial "bad girl" who leads us away from all that's right and holy. This book welcomes the return of desire like a beloved prodigal daughter.

The care and feeding of sexual desire begins with knowing what we want, when to assert our selves, and when to surrender and let go. This is the ultimate secret to great sex. It's the secret to a great life. If we could figure out how to package this understanding, we'd all be billionaires. Bon appétit!

Part One

∞

DISCOVERING *the* MANY FACES *of* SEXUAL DESIRE

REFLECTIONS

What turns you on?

We tease and talk on the phone about how we will enjoy each other later that evening. Eye contact and body language can be a great turn-on as well. The simple act of slowing down and really having a ritual sets the stage.

    —Thirty-nine-year-old cosmetician from Birmingham, Alabama

Making love outdoors in nature and the elements; role playing—elaborate erotic scenarios; sensual dance and stripping, with partner and alone; exhibitionism—watching and being watched; writing erotica and/or reading it to each other, watching romantic and sensuous movies alone and with partners; masturbating and using water with and without partners; making love on moving objects: vehicles, animals, equipment; sensual shaving of self and/or partner (whole body—but one part at a time); sensual massage of the whole body; sensual reflexology and sensual aromatherapy; bi-curiosity and fantasy . . .

    —Fifty-one-year-old housewife from Secaucus, New Jersey

Letting another person touch me emotionally as well as physically. Risking love and rejection side by side, yet sensing that there can be no real rejection—because the exploration is into the oneness between us.

    —Forty-two-year-old teacher from Syracuse, New York

1

OPENING YOURSELF TO SEXUAL DESIRE

I SEEM TO SPEND much of my professional life reassuring people that it's OK to feel good. Too many of us have been led to believe it's self-indulgent or immoral. Don't touch, don't taste, don't even think about it. Or we've learned that feeling good is all about material possessions—a glitzy ring, a flashy car. Or we imagine feeling good is about looking good. Self-esteem can sometimes hinge on a manicure. It's the joy of shopping, not the joy of sex and intimacy.

What about a larger view of feeling good—one that offers more beauty, more vitality, more sense of belonging to yourself, more connection with your partner? What about self-affirming, emotionally juicy, transformational sexual experience? I'm not talking only about sexual performance, where intercourse or orgasm becomes the goal. I'm talking about pleasure that touches your core. I'm talking about feelings that reverberate far beyond the bedroom, and positive energy that expands your whole life.

This is what I call the return of desire. It means opening yourself up. It means knowing that it really is OK to say yes to what you want—and to let go of what no longer serves you. It's the sense that feeling good sexually is a path of discovery, and an essential part of who you are. It's not about your hormone levels. It's not about measuring up to what others say. It's about *you*.

The Many Faces of Sexual Desire

Sexual desire goes by many names: attraction, passion, love, energy, libido, and randy, all-consuming lust. It can fill us with wonder. It can lift our hearts, rock our bodies, touch our souls. It involves what I call skin hunger—the longing for hot, sensual touch. It also involves the inner woman—our cravings to know and be known. It involves the loves, wishes, dreams, memories, fantasies, and meanings that are ongoing parts of our lives.

3

But sexual desire is so full of contradictions in today's culture that it's difficult to define it in an absolute way. On the one hand, sex is everywhere. Seventy-seven percent of network TV contains sexual material, says the Kaiser Family Foundation. Add to this the sexual material we encounter daily, from wolf whistles on the street to in-your-face images in commercials, billboards, rap music, the blogosphere, YouTube—you name it. Yet if you grew up in a just-say-no family or community, you probably never talked about sex, even in whispers. There was no direct language. Sexual desire was an invisible force of nature. When the winds blew right there was pleasure, life was good. Ill winds could bring darkness, pain, violation.

To complicate matters, hundreds of experts have written articles and books that frame sexual desire as a host for some grim problem—a medical syndrome, a loss of "drive," a "sexless marriage." A much-publicized paper in a 1999 issue of the *Journal of the American Medical Association* asserts that a whopping 43 percent of all American women just aren't interested in sex—this based mainly on questions about how often 1,749 of them had intercourse, but never inquiring about their emotions or the quality of their relationships. My colleague, Petra Boynton, informs me of a new desire disease on the horizon: the British are now speaking of "dating toxins"—a mix of low self-esteem, shyness, pickiness, and desperation—which are said to "infect" 5.6 million single people in the United Kingdom, preventing them from getting it on with each other or even asking each other out.

Such assertions and reports may sound silly when you stop to think about them. But there's a serious edge. The disease-based view of sexual desire is supported by science because epidemiological studies focus on dysfunction—and some of the studies are funded by the pharmaceutical companies that create the medications for the diseases. Most important, I feel, this view dictates how we judge our own intimacies, our own sexual performance. By the time the studies trickle down to most of us they're presented as breaking news. You might think low sexual desire is a national epidemic, for at times it seems to get as much press as global warming.

The truth is, fluctuations in desire do pose genuinely painful problems for many women—and their partners. For some sexual desire gets derailed. For some it goes entirely missing. "For me it's stress, boredom, and rotten relationships," complains one woman. Others cite hormonal changes, illness, or surgery. "Our sex life was devastated after my hysterectomy," says a fifty-eight-year-old teacher. Other women find desire altered by fear of pleasure, or by the antidepressants they take to relieve the fear. Still others may experience the shadow side of sexual desire—guilt, shame, abuse, violence. In the pages that follow I take all these issues seriously—as breaches of our birthright to pleasure and intimacy. At the same time, I also keep us mindful of the larger picture of health and satisfaction—so we don't stay mired in the depths of pain and dysfunction.

The Scientific View—Sex as Performance

In the mid 1960s, the sex-therapy team of William Masters and Virginia Johnson developed a model of human sexual response that quickly became the gold standard for all subsequent research in human sexuality—especially after a phase of desire was added in the late 1970s by Helen Singer Kaplan, author of *Disorders of Desire* and other books on the medical treatment of sexual dysfunction. These pioneering researchers posited that this basic medical model represented the universal pattern of sexual activity—beginning with desire, and moving phase by physiological phase through arousal and orgasm to resolution. It's worth taking a look at this model, because it has formed the basis of the way that most of us make judgments about how we carry on our sexual relationships.

I've sketched an outline of their combined sexual response cycle below. As you can see, it's a performance model—goal-oriented and focused on getting from desire to orgasm with no room for straying from the track.

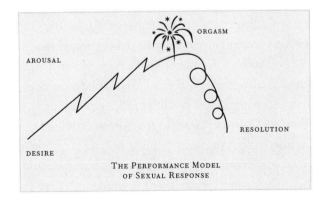

THE PERFORMANCE MODEL
OF SEXUAL RESPONSE

What is missing from this performance model of sex? For one thing, it's disconnected from the rest of life. The desire phase appears out of the blue, with no antecedent, no history. And the cycle ends when you roll over on your side and go to sleep. This leaves out most of what actually occurs in our sexual response—which will become clearer and clearer as you read women's stories throughout this book. In addition, this model is linear, an action model—which may work fine for the men who are able to proceed in a pretty much straight trajectory from desire to "doing it" to climax to dead sleep. But if you're like most women, you take a more circular sexual path, enjoying the view before and after and along the way. This will also become clear from women's stories.

All through this book I'm going to encourage you to look at your own sexual responses in a much more expansive way—that acknowledges all the dimensions of your personal experience: emotional, mental, and spiritual as well as physical. I've found that it's from this broad perspective that it's most possible to discover what may be keeping desire at bay— and most important, to discover ways to reconnect with the vitality that informs all aspects of your life.

So instead of viewing desire as a commodity, something that we're in danger of losing or missing out on, I'd like us to agree up front that sexual desire is energy—a sustainable resource that's available to all of us if we want it, even those of us who may not have it right now. Not just to lead us into steamier encounters, but to reconnect us with ourselves and our partners, and to discover new sources of pleasure and joy.

Also, if you've been searching for desire for a long time without finding it, let's consider that you may have been searching in the wrong place. Maybe you've been looking outside of yourself instead of inside. My experience as a therapist and as a human being on this planet tells me that the key to finding desire sometimes requires a deep and fearless search for yourself. You can apply to the bureau of missing persons, but if the person missing is you, you are going to have to participate fully in the search. I've had clients who've called me "the restorer of lost women to themselves." But I always decline that honor. You are the only one who can find the missing you. Let the search be part of your adventure as you read this book.

Beyond Performance—Giving Yourself Permission to Feel Good

Accepting that it's OK to feel good is a big leap for some of us—it was for me. From earliest childhood I had the job of rescuer in my alcoholic and neglectful family. It took years of failed relationships, psychotherapy, and spiritual healing before I uncovered my pleasure-loving self hiding under layers of emotional armor. When I finally emerged, I had to learn how to resonate with myself beyond pain and suffering—and beyond trying to be Superwoman. I had to learn not to rescue people who didn't want to be rescued. Most of all, maybe, I had to learn not to say no when I really wanted to say yes, yes, YES!

A defining moment dawned for me when I received my first massage—neck, back, belly, legs, the whole works. I was thirty-eight years old. When I rose glistening with oil from the table, it was the first time I ever remember being free from physical pain. The disorienting thing was that I hadn't been aware I'd been hurting—because up to then I'd been clenching every body part I could against feeling bad. In holding so tight all those years I'd also managed to keep myself from feeling a full range of pleasure. In my newly vibrant state, I realized that a significant portion of my life had simply passed me by. I'd been too numb to notice it.

As I trained to become a psychotherapist, and eventually a sex therapist, I learned I wasn't the only human being walking around only *seeming* to be present. Many of us live out our days—and nights—far removed from our deepest feelings. I now know that we develop defenses against feeling for very good reasons—so we can survive the traumas and dramas that shape our lives. But if we defend ourselves hard enough for long enough, we lose the ability to respond to new information—our systems become programmed to respond to what happened in the past rather than to what's happening in the present. So we may find our sexual relationships locked into painful patterns of repetition. It's a universal problem, but each of us has our own unique story.

If you've developed any kinds of numbness in order to survive, that pattern may still be with you, wreaking some havoc with your sexual desire. For it's not possible to feel a full longing for pleasure when you've cut yourself off from your most basic emotions and sensations. You can't open to the wonders of human connection when you're constantly recycling your old defenses against disappointment and hurt. In part 2 of this book, you can read more about these defenses—and how you might find your own ways back to "yes." But for now I want to introduce you to a model of sexuality that has proven to be a powerful tool for waking up from numbness and rediscovering sexual desire and pleasure. I call it the ISIS model.

Integrating Sexuality, Spirituality (and More)
The ISIS Wheel of Sexual Desire

In the late 1990s I conducted an independent national survey to explore questions about sexual desire that other sex researchers hadn't begun to address in an organized way. The survey questions were drawn from ones I'd been exploring with clients and colleagues over more than three decades of practice as a sex therapist: How does sex feel? What do we find most compelling and meaningful about it? What role does sexual desire play in our lives? How do we open ourselves most vibrantly to desire? How do we communicate our wishes to our partners? Does desire necessarily fizzle over the years?

The survey was titled "Integrating Sexuality and Spirituality"—ISIS for short. I know it may be unusual to see the words "sexuality" and "spirituality" next to each other. In this culture they are generally regarded as quite distinct from one another, even antithetical. Sex is understood to be primarily physical—as in the Masters-Johnson-Kaplan model above. And spirituality is understood to be intangible—and often paired with religion, which may carry with it a whole code of prohibitions about sexual behavior. Yet my research has shown that sexual and spiritual experience share a common and undeniable core quality: a hunger for connection and meaning.

Nearly four thousand people answered the ISIS survey—mostly

women, ages eighteen to eighty-six, who came from all over the country. Four in five of these respondents agreed: "For me, sex is much more than intercourse; it involves all of me—body, mind, heart, and soul." And almost half of them said they'd actually experienced a connection with "God or universal energy" at the moment of sexual ecstasy. Nearly fifteen hundred of them wrote me letters—courageous moving outpourings that reinforced my sense that desire involves far more than physical performance. Many of us long to experience a depth of sexual pleasure that can melt our boundaries and surround us with a sense of cosmic love and support.

The responses to this survey inspired me to propose an expanded model of sexual experience, which you can find in my earlier book *The Heart and Soul of Sex*. Here, I've translated it into a medicine wheel of sexual desire—a template for personal awareness and growth.

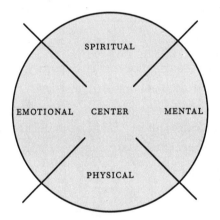

THE ISIS WHEEL OF SEXUAL DESIRE

As you can see from the diagram above, this ISIS Wheel looks very different from the physiological sexual response cycle of the earlier sex researchers. Six of the major differences will become clear in chapters that follow:

- Sexual desire is connected to the whole of our complex and perhaps complicated selves—our physical sensations, our emotional feelings, our thoughts, and our spiritual longings.

- Sexual desire is connected to our whole history—where we came from, where we are now, and what we want our sexual futures to hold for us.

- Our intimate relationships are inseparable from the rest of our lives. How we connect with them serves as a template for how we connect with all of our relationships—from family, job, and community to how we interact with the planet.

- The most powerful aphrodisiacs are not always quick fixes that come from the outside. They are information, partnership, and positive attitudes that can last our entire lives, if we want them to.

- The ISIS Wheel is not a standard by which to measure our sexual performance. It is an organizing principle that helps us gather information for ourselves, offers us a context for our stories, and provides a flexible container into which we can fit our own experiences.

- The ISIS Wheel engages us as active participants to explore the depth and breadth of our own sexual desire.

The ISIS Wheel looks simple—and on the surface it is. But individuals and couples who have used it say using it has a profound effect on their lives. Throughout this book, I'll be emphasizing the practical uses of this model, with scores of exercises to help you understand the mysteries of your sexual desire and how they relate to your life.

This whole-person, whole-life approach to sexual desire runs counter to current medical opinion, which would have us believe that balancing testosterone levels is the major answer. But in my years as a therapist and researcher I've learned that sexual desire is much more than just physical. We can't always reclaim it through prescription. Nor can we possess it through wishful thinking, power shopping, or other strategies that take us away from our selves.

What I have learned from the stories of thousands of women is that it is possible to call sexual desire into our lives with intention on the kinds of pleasure that touch your core. As you read the chapters that follow, I invite you to acknowledge your hunger to feel good, to construct your life around what's meaningful, to cultivate ways to feel powerful—not in the sense of dominating others, but in the sense that a flower is powerful when it opens. This is the power of fully expressing who you are.

Now I invite you to come with me to explore the paths of the ISIS Wheel—and the four energies that spark your sexual desire.

2

THE FOUR ENERGIES THAT SPARK SEXUAL DESIRE

ENGAGING IN THE SEARCH for your sources of sexual desire means activating all your energies of body, mind, heart, and spirit. This holds true no matter what your age or your prior history—and it may hold true even if you're not consciously aware you're activating them. In *The Heart and Soul of Sex*, I've written extensively about these four energies, and I'll review them here, with a focus on how they spark your sexual desire. If you refer to the diagram in chapter 1, you'll see that these energies are all part of the ISIS Wheel. Let's look at each one of them now, as if we can walk right into the ISIS Wheel—starting with the physical path.

Physical Energy
The Path of Sensation

The kinds of activities we most often associate with sexual desire are physical. And these activities are generally associated with sexual performance—that is, genital touching and intercourse with a goal of orgasm. In our culture, this is the so-called "real thing."

But if you listen closely to women speak about what really turns them on, most say their physical appetites aren't limited only to genital stimulation—what one woman calls "zeroing in on the homing sites." Though homing-site contact may feel pretty wonderful, it can feel even better when you connect these few parts of you with the rest of you so they don't feel so isolated. The truth is, our whole bodies cry out to be touched. We want hugging, kissing, massage, a sensuous bath—many women say all-over touching *is* the real thing. For some "all-over" ideas see the Extragenital Matrix in the back of this book. This is a simple touch grid I developed to suggest how we can explore delicious sensations on many receptive parts of our bodies.

But let's not stop at touch. The path of physical sensation includes more. Seeing, tasting, smelling—these can also spark sexual desire. One of the women who answered the ISIS survey describes the sensual power of hearing. She says that Beethoven is what originally did it for her. At a fateful moment a number of years ago, she happened to experience a five-star orgasm while she was listening to the choral finale of the Ninth Symphony, the *Ode to Joy*. Since then, music has become an ever-ready turn-on for her—when she's with her partner, and also when she's alone.

But beyond Beethoven, and even beyond music, the whole world can act as your sensual playground. One woman sums it up:

> To me sexuality is not based on intercourse . . . All creative acts and the power of nature is sexual energy. Swimming in the ocean is erotic. Watching a lovely sunset is erotic. Eating a juicy sweet peach is erotic.

Physical desire resides in how we move in our bodies, too—our pleasure in breathing, stretching, dancing, undulating our bellies, and swaying our hips—especially in resonance with a partner. All these can affect us deeply and open us to erotic sensation even though they aren't directly focused on genital performance. The movement pioneer who has guided me to explore some of these subtle avenues to desire is Emilie Conrad, author of *Life on Land* and creator of Continuum, a uniquely fluid method of breathing and moving that she teaches all over the world.

Physical desire wakes us up—and the body doesn't stop at the skin, as Conrad regularly points out in her teaching. Our physical desires involve our minds, emotions, and spirits, too. In the words of one of the respondents of the ISIS survey, "The heart becomes smoothed and stroked as well."

Physical desire also resides in our relationships. It resides in our ability to create excitement, beauty, comfort, a safe haven for each other. It resides in intelligent touch—where you and your partner set out to know every inch and fold of each other. It resides in permission to let go of the image of the perfect body we're all taught to strive for—reminding us to relax our shoulders, bellies, buttocks, jaws, and all the body parts we tend to clench tight during our day jobs. Sometimes familiarity is what does it for us. Sometimes what's irresistible is a new lover with a new perspective and a new touch. One woman says she never found this permission in her twelve-year marriage, but her current sweetheart encourages her to "open and flower" during lovemaking—"I can yell or be loud, look into his eyes at orgasm, masturbate, or bring myself pleasure."

Another woman expresses her experience of physical energy on the path of sensation as poetry in motion.

> My body knows the sweetness and glory
> Of the language your hand whispers to it.
> Like a waking child
> My body recognizes you—
> Your touch finds its way
> To the secret places of my body
> And whispers again to my soul.

Emotional Energy
The Path of Passion and Compassion

Emotional energy is as integral to sexual desire as physical energy is—and it's almost as palpable. This is the path of passion and compassion; of love, caring, and empathy; of safety, power, and pleasure. Women speak of melting into intimacy with their lovers. Of feeling filled with sweetness as well as lust.

Our emotional energy can be a powerful initiator into sexual desire. "An affirmation," says an Indiana social worker. "Sharing our passion of life," says a designer from West Virginia. "We have an intense deep love for each other that has seen us through many hardships—it is the tie that binds us totally," writes a humanities teacher. "With my partner, I mean, WOW!" effuses a grateful abuse survivor who says her present lover represents a U-turn from her long history of rape, alcoholism, and divorce. For her, the essentials of sexual desire are caring and nurturing—the ability to give as well as receive. Also essential is her self-esteem—the sense that she can value herself and her own wishes—and discover a new capacity for empathy—the sensitivity to appreciate her partner's feelings, wants, and needs.

I've heard woman after woman assert that there's a vast difference between just having physical sex and *making love*—with a full range of affection and concern for each other. The emotional energy of desire informs all the components of lovemaking—eye contact, heart contact, laughter, and words that touch the core. For some women, these words are "sweet nothings"—praise, romantic love talk, and poetry, delivered with warmth and focused attention. For others, the words may be earthy and explicit rather than sugar-sweet. (If earthy happens to be your thing and you want suggestions on how to move beyond a few four-letter clichés, read Sallie Tisdale's wonderful book *Talk Dirty to Me* and Aline Zold-brod's *Sex Talk*.)

But the emotions of desire include many intangibles, too—and scientists are beginning to recognize these as they use sophisticated imaging equipment to investigate the psychoneurobiology of love. Anthropologist Helen Fisher (*Why We Love*) and her colleagues at Rutgers University have been able to document in the laboratory that love is a potent aphrodisiac—and far more effective than ginseng, oysters, or the fabled ground rhinoceros horn. It's more eco-friendly too, because it's a constantly renewable resource.

Brain scans of love-struck college students reveal that love literally lights us up—that is, it lights up the deepest, darkest, most primitive regions of our brains. When these regions are activated, they affect other regions of the brain as well, including those that control our thoughts and emotions. Brain scans of these students also reveal how love enhances the sensuous ways of dopamine, a neurotransmitter that triggers exhilaration, focused attention, and motivation for reward. But God forbid you should feel rejected. Hormonal activity may be even more intense when love is withdrawn, say Fisher and company. You may be subject to rage, revenge, suicidal depression, and worse.

All this is groundbreaking twenty-first-century information. But it's also very old news. Over the centuries poets and artists and just plain women have exalted the wings-on-your-heels pleasures of romantic love—and also the dark emotions that haunt us when we get left in the lurch. "Hell hath no fury like a woman scorned," wrote playwright William Congreve some three hundred years ago, echoing sentiments from the ancient Greek poet Sappho to our own contemporary Eve Ensler, author of *The Vagina Monologues,* a performance piece that has raised global awareness of both sexual pleasure and abuse.

Mental Energy
The Path of Discernment

We use our mental energy to help us make decisions about what we want. We use it to ask questions: Who am I and who am I attracted to—men, women, or both? Am I really monogamous—or do I crave the variety of more than one partner? What is sex anyway? Is it really all about inter-course for me? Is there something more? Am I in step with everybody else—or two-stepping to my own rhythm? Am I through with all those exhausting mating rituals and happy to be alone and celibate?

We use our mental energy to field the conflicting messages that come at us from everywhere—e-mail, TV, glossy ads in which women's body parts are used to sell everything from beer to sports cars. We also use it to sort through the messages we've received our whole lives long—"Good girls don't." "Real men score." "If you really loved me you'd . . ." These are the kinds of phrases that reverberate from locker-room conversa-tions, religious instruction, our mothers' advice, and more. They all add up—and they influence our sexual desire in the here and now. Think how your life might be different if you'd had access to accurate information about sex when you were growing up. Or if you'd been given positive, age-appropriate counseling about how to ask for what you wanted—body, mind, heart, and spirit? Chances are your sexual thoughts and dreams would be clearer of negative criticism and judgments—and that you could more gracefully discern what you want now and who you want to do it with.

Our mental energy is active during our dreams, fantasies, and other flights of sexual imagination. And as a therapist, I'm constantly reminded how profoundly our sexual desire is affected by our memories. It's con-nected to flashbacks of past lovemaking—the good, the bad, and the ugly.

It's connected to the books we read and films we see. The desire for sexual connection doesn't begin when we're already in the bedroom, socks off and door bolted. And it doesn't end when we roll off each other's bodies and sink into a torporous sleep. It's intimately connected to the whole sweep of our daily lives—the thousand details of living that inform our sexual pleasure, where doing the dishes can register as high on the Richter scale as a gift of red roses.

Spiritual Energy
The Path of Connection and Meaning

Sexual desire is intricately linked with reaching out to find meaning in our lives, whether that's affirmation, or love, or liberation, or a sense of connection with nature and the divine. These are what transpersonal psychiatrist Carl Jung calls the "irrational facts of experience." You can't count them or measure them, but they're always present. It's a matter of opening yourself enough to be aware of them.

Connecting sexual and spiritual energy is at the core of personal vitality and well-being, say thousands of women who responded to my ISIS survey. They say this connection leads to "freedom and joyous play," "life force," and "divine connection"—that is, to experiences that may radiate far beyond the bedroom to energize their whole lives. This merging of sexual and spiritual energy can recharge relationships, enhance self-esteem, transform belief systems, and heal mind and body after histories of disappointment and abuse.

"When I looked into his eyes," says one ISIS respondent, "I felt a rush as if a piece of my soul had joined his and been left with him for safe keeping. He felt it too." It's not always that easy, though. Another woman recounts her ongoing struggle to connect sex and spirit—and surrender to desire.

> There have been numerous times where my strong spiritual nature has battled with my equally strong sexuality. However, when they combine during love my spirit soars, often leaving me with an intense joy that my body cannot always contain.

Spontaneous tears of deep, pure emotion come forth—much akin to the tears of overwhelming spiritual joy at my children's births.

For these women and many others, there's a significant "Oh God!" factor in sexual desire. As I explained in chapter 1, I'm not talking about religion necessarily, but about the basic human desire for connection and meaning. These women consistently talk about experience that's way beyond physical orgasm—the kind that opens us to deeper connections with ourselves, our partners, and a power beyond ourselves—God, Goddess, nature, waterfall, or whatever we choose to name it.

Some women enter into sex worshipfully. For them, sexual desire may arise through ceremonies or rituals that focus sacred intention—meditation, prayer, flowers, candles, incense, bathing, special foods. Some women engage in Tantric practices to develop intimate and sensual bonds with their partners and also with spirit. Tantra is an ancient practice that's gaining increasing popularity in the present—for more information, check out the scores of books and millions of websites, including www.tantra.com, and also see my chapter on Tantra in *The Heart and Soul of Sex*.

But even without a specialized practice you can open to the spiritual essence of your sexual desire. A longtime survivor of abuse, addiction, and guilt says her desire is a spiritual experience in and of itself:

> I literally vibrate with the energies that are inside of me. I feel above the earth, my senses are heightened, and I have increased stamina. When we share orgasms, I feel that we are "touching souls." To me, my body really is a temple, and spiritual sex (or sex of any kind) is the most pure form of worship that I can practice.

When the Four Energies Merge
The Center of the Wheel

Much of our experience of sexual desire takes place at the perimeter of the ISIS Wheel—it leads to a hug or kiss, or a bit of canoodling when you're too tired to be fully frisky. But sometimes sexual desire plunges us directly into the center—a place of compelling physical sensations, of emotional, mental, and spiritual transformation.

The center of the ISIS Wheel is the place where all four of our energies merge. Here, we connect with the physical aspect of desire—our bodies flow with sensation. We connect with the emotional aspect of desire— our hearts expand with love and compassion. We connect with the mental aspect of desire—our imaginations flood with light and color and memory. We connect with the spiritual aspect of desire—we enter a vibrant terrain of feeling and being. As an artist from New York describes it, "It's the sense of oneness with my partner and the universe. The calm and peacefulness. Overcoming the barriers of fear so we could just be one in the moment."

Only you can describe the specific details of how you experience this landscape of the center. Many women say they can't find adequate words— not surprising because our language of sexual desire has been so focused on the performance aspects of sex. It may help you to begin with images rather than words. If you are willing, you can practice finding your own images right now—by remembering times when your energies merged in the center. I prefer to spell this "re-membering," to convey the notion that all the information we need to know about sexual desire is already there at some deep layer of our consciousness—all we have to do is give it substance.

Re-Membering the Center

Remember a time when you experienced sexual ecstasy—or pleasure, or orgasm. These are your positive "re-runs," as one of my research mentors used to say. Or you can remember any delicious experience you've had, whether it's overtly sexual or not.

Be still, be comfortable, be open, and notice how your body responds as you bask in this delicious experience. Does your breathing deepen? Does your jaw relax? Does tension drain from your shoulders and pelvis? Does your heart feel lighter? These are some of the responses I notice in my body.

Many women say their minds fill with light or with music. Other women say their hearts fill with love for their partners. One woman describes this as "times in which the body/spirit sings." Another says she was flooded with fragrance that took her to "the botanical gardens of heaven." Another woman says it was physical sensation that inundated her as she remembered caressing her naked body as she lay on a flat rock one lazy summer afternoon:

> The sun beat down on my skin, birds sang, wind shook the trees, and fluffy clouds carried away worries, cares, and concerns as I came with the power greater than self . . . God (she has so many titles these days).

As you allow yourself to fill with positive memories of your sensual, sexual self, your whole energy field will grow larger, more vibrant. Brain researchers can actually measure these changes. This energetic expansion changes you, and if you're in a relationship it can change your relationship, too. When you expand in this way, your energy field stimulates your partner's to expand and brighten, as well.

You may be able to feel the energy exchanges between you and your partner as an electric tingling or buzzing in your hands and feet—"as if my life battery is charging," says one woman. Or you may feel them in your heart—as a surge of love and desire for connection. You may feel them pulsing in your lips or breasts or genitals, or a streaming sensation up and down your spine, or a melting of your pelvis and uterus—the varieties are endless.

Some women recognize this flow of sexual energy and welcome it. For other women it can feel scary, extraordinary, or even weird. "Is it normal for me to feel these things?" But many women find it difficult to feel much energy flowing at all. In the next chapter you'll see why. Your four energies of sexual desire can go underground when they meet the kinds of rigid scripts the mainstream culture gives us. You'll learn what we're all taught desire is supposed to be like, and how you're supposed to fit your sexual feelings into a cultural box that's far too small. You'll also find keys to help you open the cultural box so that you can reclaim your sexual desire on your own terms.

3

WHAT'S "NORMAL"?

Reviewing Your Scripts about Sexual Desire

As YOU BEGIN to explore your own paths to sexual desire, you may find yourself encountering a widespread assumption in today's world: "normal" is equated with successful and frequent intercourse. This is a cripplingly narrow definition for many women—because as you've already seen, sexual desire can expand far beyond how well you perform. It also includes how you feel, how you think, and what sex means to you, to your relationships, and to your life.

Though most of us aren't aware of it, we each carry some carefully crafted internal scripts about how sex is supposed to be—a story about what's right, what's hot, and what's not. We carry these scripts in our minds of course, and many of us can recite them chapter and verse. But we also carry them in our bodies—they show up in how fluidly or painfully we move, or how open or defended we are in our intimate contact. We carry these scripts in our total energy field, too—in our emotional and spiritual longings for pleasure and connection—or our rejections of feeling good.

Usually our scripts of sexual desire are laid down early in our lives—passed on to us by our parents, our community, our peers, and our culture. Too often, we never stop to look at the scripts, or question that our sexual desire may be motivated by something other than, well, sexual desire. In this chapter I'll discuss four scripts that regularly limit the flow of sexual desire in our bodies, hearts, minds, and spirits. These are the performance script, the romantic love script, the good-girl script, and the script I describe by the exclamation, "Oh God!"

The Performance Script

The performance script centers on intercourse and orgasm. And because these activities are easy to study and measure, sex researchers have focused an immense amount of attention on every nuance. In fact, most sex research follows the classic performance script: how much, how many, with whom—ranging from arousal to orgasm to G-spot ejaculation. If your desire for sex doesn't live up to this script, it's framed as a dysfunction—or, as today's sex therapists prefer, a "disorder." But whatever way you slice it, dysfunction or disorder means somebody thinks there's something wrong with you.

The performance script is stoutly reinforced by definitions in the American Psychiatric Association's *Diagnostic and Statistical Manual of Mental Disorders* used by health professionals who treat sexual problems. In this *DSM,* the criteria for sexual dysfunction are all physical, and they all relate specifically to problems with intercourse. This means that the term "desire disorder" doesn't officially refer to erotic feelings or interest in sexual relationship. It only means lack of interest in the act of penis-vagina intercourse.

Let me point out that there is a giant double message in the reasoning regarding this issue. While the medical criteria for sexual dysfunction are focused on intercourse, at the same time at least two generations of sex researchers have consistently reported that some three-quarters of women are not actually satisfied by intercourse. These reports maintain that we need clitoral stimulation, along with extended warm-up periods of so-called foreplay.

There are other flaws in the *DSM* mind-set, too. For instance, not all women have partners to have intercourse with. Not all partnered women have male partners to have intercourse with—or male partners who are able to perform the act of intercourse. And not all women choose intercourse as their favorite sexual activity even if they do have eagerly performing male partners. But here's the major rub: even if women are highly motivated by sexual activities that don't include intercourse—like clitoral stimulation or oral sex, for instance—they can be diagnosed by the book as dysfunctional—because they're not panting for intercourse. So is this dysfunction? Or is the *DSM* dysfunctional? Either way, it leaves out an essential truth I hear from women all over the country: that there's a great deal more to sex than intercourse.

All of that said, let's have a look at what science says our performance disorders are about, and how we should go about fixing them—by the book.

TESTOSTERONE, ESTROGEN, AND DHEA, OH MY!

The medicalizing of sexual desire is a hot-button issue today. Prescriptions for pills, creams, and hormone-releasing patches are sought by countless women in the hopes that these will jump-start their interest in intercourse. An especially big player is testosterone, which is widely hyped as "the hormone of desire." While this book doesn't promote a medical approach to increasing your sexual desire (the research and exercises here go way beyond the medical model), it's important to acknowledge at the outset that some women do have hormone imbalances. If you are one of these women, your biology really may be your destiny as Sigmund Freud suggested some hundred years ago. Balancing your hormone levels may activate a seemingly magical return of desire, at least for a while. However, be aware that over time testosterone can also trigger some unwanted side effects. Will you grow a beard? Will you be singing bass in your church choir? For the lurid details read Paul Joannides's irreverently researched *Guide to Getting It On*.

Much of the literature on hormones is written persuasively, and with the stamp of medical prescription. But even some physicians argue that hormone intervention for sexual desire is not the only way. For one thing, the science of hormone use is inexact. There's no consensus among physicians about how to measure or interpret your high or low hormone levels, nor is there certainty about what the effects might be on your particular body.

And there are inherent contradictions. Some women with high testosterone levels report low sexual desire, and some women with low levels report high sexual desire. In a heated discussion on a professional electronic mailing list I belong to, one physician colleague reports "dramatic success" in treating women with regularly monitored testosterone, especially in combination with estrogen, progesterone, and DHEA, a hormone that stimulates the adrenals. Another colleague counters: "There is not a single study that shows endogenous testosterone levels to be correlated with female sexual interest in partnered sex." Still another colleague says, "One can read the testosterone data according to one's own frame of reference. It's like explaining the Bible according to one's own belief."

How do you know if hormone treatment might be right for you? Let's say your desire dropped suddenly—as if a light switch were flicked off, say some women. And let's say there's no reason you can name for this sudden drop, such as divorce, illness, job loss, a disgruntled teenager tyrannizing your household, or other such stressors. And let's say your relationship is great and that you have a positive self-image, no history of abuse, no underlying depression, no diabetes, no autoimmune problems, no metabolic imbalances. And you're eating properly, exercising regularly, generally managing your stress, and you're not living next to a toxic waste site. When you run out of factors like these as possible reasons for your drop in desire, then you might consider hormone intervention.

But you can't really determine whether hormones will restore lost libido until you try them. Prudent doctors advise a trial period. And they add, "Proceed with caution." If you want to pursue the hormonal roots of your desire, there is a great deal of information available—on the Internet and also in some notable books. These include *The Hormone of Desire* by psychiatrist Susan Rako, and *For Women Only*, by the Berman sisters— Jennifer (a urologist) and Laura (a sex therapist, and director of her own clinic in Chicago).

If you want to explore more holistic and "natural" hormonal approaches to sexual desire, check out the Alexander Foundation for Women's Health on the Internet (www.afwh.org) and read Christiane Northrup's wise books, *Women's Bodies, Women's Wisdom*, and *The Wisdom of Menopause*. *Our Bodies, Ourselves*, the classic guide for women of all ages, added a splendidly researched new volume in 2006: *Our Bodies, Ourselves, Menopause*. The Resources section points to other places you can pursue specific questions you have about hormone treatments.

"FEMALE SEXUAL DYSFUNCTION"
AN INVENTED DISEASE?

To add to the confusion about hormones and sexual desire, much of today's hormone research is funded by pharmaceutical companies—the very ones that create the products that doctors prescribe to cure sexual dysfunction. Even a rookie investigator can see that this makes for researcher bias on a flagrant scale. It gives corporations the potential to dictate the criteria for women's sexual health rather than responding to the needs and wishes of women.

With this scenario in mind, some prominent social scientists, physicians, and health care providers around the country have gone on record to say they think female sexual dysfunction (FSD) is, at least in part, a disease conjured up by Big Pharma to generate sales. Feminist psychologist and researcher Leonore Tiefer is the leading spirit behind an innovative watchdog organization called the New View Campaign, which collaborates with other savvy public health advocacy organizations like the National Women's Health Network and Our Bodies Ourselves to challenge the notion that drugs are the magic fix for low sexual desire. A New View tenet is that desire is complex and there are myriad reasons for low sexual desire besides hormone imbalances. These reasons include lack of sex education, lack of health care, clueless lovers, abuse, and poverty—to name just a few.

But these reasons for low libido don't figure in the medical view, where the approach is not designed to relieve the causes but to provide a quick fix for symptoms. Since the blockbuster debut of Viagra in 1998, the pharmaceutical industry has worked to create a market for a pink Viagra—to make women randy for all the men on blue Viagra. One such "pink" product is Procter & Gamble's proposed Intrinsa patch. This patch, to be worn like a Band-Aid, is designed to release a steady supply of testosterone into the bloodstream, and keep its wearers constantly on the brink of lust. But at what price? The gnarly fact downplayed by P&G is that Intrinsa's side effects include strokes and heart attacks. In December 2004, the New View helped block FDA approval for its marketing in the United States—though Intrinsa is presently available in Europe.

Stepford Vaginas
A twenty-first-century fashion statement?

New View members also discuss the negative implications of genital surgery on sexual desire. These surgeries include the ritual puberty rites of female genital cutting (FGC), or female genital mutilation (FGM), which is the term originally coined by the World Health Organization. These rites have been practiced in a number of cultures for centuries—for the express purpose of controlling sexual activity in girls and women, and branding them for ownership by their eventual husbands. For an inimitable journey through the agonies of genital mutilation and its aftermath, read Alice Walker's *Possessing the Secret of Joy*.

Now, in America, there's a new wrinkle—highly advertised genital enhancement surgeries, often termed "vaginal rejuvenation." You can go online and find a plastic surgeon to snip and shape your genitals to make you conform to somebody else's standards of beauty. God forbid your labia might not be symmetrical. Or that your "down there" doesn't look exactly like every other woman's. It's a message worthy of the classic sci-fi movie *The Body Snatchers*, or maybe *The Stepford Wives*, where suburban housewives' brains are replaced by computer chips that tell them how to conform to their hubbies' ideas of perfection.

If you surf the Internet for information, you'll find thousands of entries for cosmetic vaginal surgery—or so-called "designer vaginas." You can try "LabiaDoctor.com." Or "Dr. Blatt Repairs Labia and Tightens Vagina." Or try TheGShot.com. The latest surgical intervention for a problem we never knew we had is called the "G Shot." This is an injection of collagen into the anterior of your vaginal wall to enlarge your G spot. The advertised effect is to enhance sexual pleasure, but so far the jury is out on whether it generates pleasure or pain. One New View colleague exclaims, "Ouch!" Another points out, "This is FGM, American Style." You can find more such information on the New View website, www.fsd-alert.org, and also in the book edited by Tiefer and Ellyn Kaschak, *A New View of Women's Sexual Problems*.

Lest you be tempted to pursue genital surgery as an antidote to low desire, here's something these ads don't tell you: every woman's vulva is as distinctive as her facial features. If you want to check this out for yourself, get together with a bunch of friends some weekend and have a look at how individual your various vaginal lips and clitorises are. See if you follow the current fashion of shaving and sculpting your pubic hair or if you leave it *au naturelle*. If this feels too down home and personal, there are colorful books of vulva photographs, including Joani Blank's *Femalia* and Nick Karras's *Petals*. In his beautiful book *The Yoni: Sacred Symbol of Female Creative Power*, Dutch researcher Rufus Camphausen shows how our vulvas are reflected in history and nature. An added benefit of paying this kind of attention to an often hidden aspect of yourself may be that it's just what you need to spark new sexual interest.

EXPLORING PHYSICAL DESIRE ON YOUR OWN TERMS

As you can see, the performance script is limiting and maybe physically harmful. So we need to find other approaches that invite our bodies to open up to sexual desire and pleasure.

Take a few moments right now to explore the physical aspect of desire in your life. Do you love how you look—or do you criticize yourself? When your partner wants to cuddle, do you open up in anticipation—or do you tense up? What feels good to you—is there warmth, excitement, lubrication? What feels not so good—do you experience vaginal pain, dryness, or muscle spasms that prevent you from opening to the pleasure you desire?

In the following chapters you'll see many physical approaches to exploring and reclaiming your sexual desire. These include breathing, bathing, floating, touching, and visualizing. You'll read about how women use vibrators and how they exercise their pelvic floor muscles. You'll learn how you can conduct what I call "vagina dialogues" with yourself (after the *Vagina Monologues,* with apologies to Eve Ensler) so that you know what turns you on "down there"—and all over your body. All of these are designed to help you appreciate your body intelligence—the understanding that physical pleasure is connected to all aspects of your being.

The Romantic Love Script

Now let's explore the path of the emotions. According to the fairy tales we grew up on, it's all about romance. Two people fall in love and live happily and sexily ever after, with never a moment of concern about who takes out the trash. For most of us, this just isn't how it works. While this script may sound like a certain kind of ideal to strive for, it doesn't begin to tell the whole story of how our sexual emotions play out in our lives. The romance script can create unrealistic expectations that leave many of us feeling like misfits. Even worse, it can leave us in the lurch, and sometimes seriously hurt.

"My first sexual experience was date rape," writes a psychotherapist who says she still suffers from a broken heart. She finally fell in love with a "passionate, sexy man" only to find that he was cheating on her several times a week. "This betrayal was absolutely devastating. It affected my whole outlook on intimacy and sex. I have doubts that I'll ever trust enough to have that same connection." The bottom line for her: "Sex hurts—it's a chore."

Years of hearing similar stories from women has taught me that the emotional dimension of sexual desire is not all about hearts and flowers. It can also be a path of guilt and shame, of anger, fear, disgust, blame, and self-blame. It's on the path of the emotions that we meet many of the ravages of trauma and abuse. I cannot count the number of clients who live with so much rage and terror that it seems impossible for them to open up their bodies to feel sensation or open their hearts to feel love. Or like the therapist above, to feel that sex is nothing but hard work.

The fear of painful emotions can cause us to avoid sex altogether or to numb ourselves or even dissociate during sexual interactions. As one woman puts it: "Sometimes I make myself invisible—I hide under a rock and quit breathing." If this sounds like your story, you're not alone. Other women have been there, too, and some of the men in my practice have been there as well. We'll look into this dynamic in chapter 11, which explores the impact of trauma and abuse on sexual desire.

For some women an especially big desire-killer is fear of their own anger—as yet another expression of "good girls don't." If you're holding on to big anger, it's impossible to let go fully into desire—and that's true if you're suppressing your anger by medicating it into oblivion. Releasing anger can actually act as a kind of aphrodisiac, because it frees up your total energy. I'm not suggesting you lay waste to your personal landscape by yelling and screaming at your partner or anyone else. There are ways of releasing anger without frontal attack or blame. A bioenergetic approach is to beat pillows. Or you can invite your partner to join you in breaking bottles at your local landfill. For more subtle suggestions, see Harriet Lerner's classic book, *The Dance of Anger*. If you carry a level of rage that won't let go, that indicates you can use some professional support and help—see the Resources section for suggestions on how to find a therapist.

Then there are couples like George and Martha in *Who's Afraid of Virginia Woolf*, whose desire is actually fueled by sarcasm and knock-down fights. There can be a price to pay for this kind of acting out, though. I'm remembering a colleague who says she carried a load of rage from her childhood abuse and early sexual relationships. She says she used anger "like a drug" to trigger sexual lust in her lackluster first marriage.

> Anger allowed me to be highly sexual. If I did not want to be sexual, my husband would keep at me and at me and I'd work into a rage and that was the only way I could have sexual feeling. My heart would race, I'd feel invincible—as if I could do anything. The anger would hold me in the physical act. Otherwise, I'd be sick and disgusted and not engage in sex at all.

This desire-anger link gave her permission to engage in a sub-rosa kind of battering that would never make it into the police reports, but it was domestic violence nonetheless.

> When I was feeling sexual physically, I was feeling rage emotionally. My head was saying one thing and my body was saying another. My satisfaction was to withhold from him—to have physical sex without giving my whole self. I used my body as a weapon and directed the violence toward him.

"Did you come to orgasm?" I asked.

"I could come to orgasm—if I wanted. Or I could fake orgasm."

In other words, she used her own anger to arouse her sexual excitement. She also used it to create a sexual situation in which she could feel some measure of power over her husband. By controlling him sexually, she also felt as if she was getting back at the lineup of abusive men who'd preceded him in her life. Do I need to say that her marriage ended in a cloud of dust? The good news is that this was over two decades ago and my colleague is now an accomplished therapist, after years of her own emotional rehab—and she's been able to transform her negative experiences into a finely honed ability to help women who present with similar problems.

Exploring emotional desire on your own terms

So we see that the romantic love script can limit our ability for whole-person sexual desire and sometimes keep us locked into relationships that should have ended long ago. How do you assess your own feelings of desire? Do you feel open-hearted—or constricted? In terms of partnership, do you feel like reaching out for love—or like recoiling? Or like my colleague above, do your emotional turn-ons arise from a sense of getting even? When you're in bed together, do you feel a glow of warmth that draws you to one another—or an icy tension that forces you to opposite edges of the mattress?

As this book progresses, you'll find exercises on exploring and sharing deep feelings—and appreciating your partner's feelings, even if they happen to be different from yours. You'll find suggestions on how to recognize your sexual rights and how to give yourself affirmations. You'll find suggestions on how to ask for what will help make sex more alive and satisfying, whether it's eye contact, heart contact, or that indefinable something called "being present." You'll also find suggestions for sex therapy, recovery groups, support groups, and healing for traumatic experiences—including ways to release anger so that it doesn't perpetuate an endless cycle of sexual violence.

The Good-Girl Script

Now let's explore the mental path of sexual desire—where we are beset by negative judgments. Many of us are dogged throughout our lives by a voice that tells us to be a good girl. And what is that exactly? For one thing, a good girl isn't a woman who loves sex. For another, she's all about pleasing others. She conforms to dress codes. She is polite. She lets her partner take the choicest morsels on the plate. She is never "shrill." A self-described "family peacekeeper" says she still resonates to messages she got growing up in a repressive small-town household, and they still undermine her sexual self-esteem and her desire.

> I was taught to be ashamed of my body—and that it is not all
> right for a single woman to desire sexual pleasure for any rea-

son. NEVER PLEASURE. I cannot seem to rid myself of that guilt/shame, and the "you aren't doing it right" voice.

Which raises an intriguing question: How can sexual desire flourish in a culture that floods you with the message "Good girls *don't*"? How can you stay warm and cozy and seductive when your partner exclaims, "Waddaya mean—are you nuts to want something like *that*?" How can you keep desire alive when your main goal is to please others? When you have the sense that if only you were better, or thinner, or blonder, or sexier, or anything but who you really are . . . he wouldn't leave you. Or he wouldn't hit you. Or he wouldn't kill you. The papers are full of gruesome domestic murders—and of women who are considered to be fair game. It doesn't seem to matter whether your partner is an unemployed laborer or a million-dollar surgeon.

Despite the odds, some women are able to reach adulthood believing they're safe, powerful, and worthy, sexually and spiritually whole. "I was fortunate enough to grow up in a home with no religion," writes a happily partnered musician. "The only 'should' I got around sex was that I shouldn't have sex with someone I wasn't in love with."

This parental caveat about being in love is obviously well-meant and well-taken. But it raises yet another question about who gets to define our sexual desire. In some families, love and marriage are supposed to go together like the proverbial horse and carriage. But it doesn't always work out that way. Love—and certainly sex—can peter out after life intervenes with its myriad responsibilities. And sometimes it really is empowering to engage in sexual activity just for the fun of it, with no long-term strings attached.

Even a *lack* of sexual messages can dampen our sexual desire. Some of us received no information at all—for good girls are also innocent. What we don't know won't hurt us, the saying goes. This was my story. I came of age in the avoidant 1950s, before the sexual revolution, before the Internet, before sex made it openly into magazines or onto television. When I began training as a family therapist in the early 1970s, the subject of sex wasn't included in the family therapy books—even in the indexes, under "S." This led me to dive headlong into a murky void—not only to learn about my own responses but also to help the many clients I saw presenting with sexuality issues, for none of my colleagues was trained to address them. That I'd turn out to be an outspoken sexologist was clearly not what my proper Bostonian forebears had imagined for me.

EXPLORING DESIRE BY OPENING YOUR MIND

Positive thinking expands our options. At the end of the day, we all have to find our own ways to move beyond the screwy messages we got—and get—about sexual desire. As this book progresses, you'll find practical exercises to help you move beyond the good-girl script to make sense of your personal history of sexual desire. You'll find suggestions for telling your story, listening to others, reading, fantasizing, and being playful. You'll also find affirmations you can use to remind yourself that feeling good is healthy and natural, and ultimately good for the planet, too.

The chapters that follow are inspired by women who've found ways to open up their minds and trust their intuition, allow their imaginations to play, and connect with the deep wisdom in their dreams and daydreams. All these are crucial to the art of feeling good. When you can let go of judgments about what you *should* want and what sex should be like, a whole new universe can open up.

The "Oh God!" Script

This script is about the spiritual aspects of sexual desire. On the one hand, it says that if you're "doing it right" you'll feel a profound connection with your partner and you'll reach mystical heights. While much of my research and writing has been about exploring the spiritual dimension of sexuality, this information can become a burden if we hold it as yet another goal we have to live up to.

On the other hand, I've heard many women complain of feeling disconnected from sexual desire—of feeling depressed, disoriented, dissociated, or isolated from their partners. I often frame these as spiritual issues, especially if they cannot be attributed to specific incidences, such as illness or childbirth or partner abuse. They become part of those "irrational facts of experience" Carl Jung talks about. It's the downside of the "Oh God!" script—meaning that you've had it with sex—you can't deal with it anymore.

"The sexual act was hurtful, hateful, and very painful," murmurs a sexual abuse survivor. Another says, "I felt I had to have sex, with no mental or emotional connection, whenever my partner decided to feel a base need." Still another admits, "I get physically drawn into sex, but then feel emotionally detached—I'm doing shopping lists in my head."

Some women say their sexual responses feel entirely out of balance—even sometimes bizarre. A woman in recovery from substance abuse puts it this way:

> After years of trying to please the "man," I felt cheated and used. I had no close physical or spiritual feelings with my first husband of fourteen years. I would cover my head with a pillow and laugh until he had finished.

It doesn't work to try to heal a spiritual desire issue with physical or behavioral methods. A sense of essential loneliness will never be filled by testosterone supplementation. The sense of needing to cover your head and laugh until he's done will never be relieved by your being sent home to practice different positions for intercourse. Clients will almost certainly resist these assigned "homeplay" tasks by not doing them. Or they'll use them to pick fights with one another. Or they'll simply stop coming to therapy.

If you experience these sorts of disconnection, it may mean you're removing yourself from your partner, or from some past painful event that's triggered by sexual feeling. Or, as sometimes turns out, it may simply be a sign of our times. For disconnecting from sexual feeling is not always about numbing our pain. It's also about distraction. We're actually training ourselves to disconnect whenever we engage in multitasking—for instance at the gym when we exercise our bodies on the treadmill while our minds are absorbed in the talk show we're watching on TV.

Certain negative relationship dynamics feed into sexual disconnection and loneliness. These include blame and self-blame, the need to dominate a partner, and also the need to be subordinate. I'm not talking about the kinds of sexual back-and-forth that excite interest and desire—such as consensual teasing, and fantasies of delicious conquest. Nor am I talking about the power plays in consciously S/M relationships—a sexual lifestyle that aficionados say may be deeply spiritual as it stretches them so far beyond their comfort zones.

The desire-killing dynamics I'm talking about are the kinds of power discrepancies that create distress, harden the heart, constrict the body, and block sexual intimacy. The ravages of abuse and trauma litter the spiritual path of desire as well as the paths of body, heart, and mind. And when the spirit is damaged, our capacity for sexual desire suffers too. One client phrased it poignantly. She said she felt as if the song was gone from her life—and she wanted it back.

EXPLORING SPIRITUAL DESIRE ON YOUR OWN TERMS

When you look at your sexual desire from a spiritual perspective, are you moved to embrace new experiences—or do you tend to shrink back from the unknown? Do you sense fluidity and connection—or are you mainly aware of the grim lessons to be learned from sexual pain and suffering? Sexual desire is complex, and most of us experience an intricate combination of both. I've often found that it's only when we can dive deep enough into our pool of pain that we can find our way to pleasure. And that sometimes we can literally reframe pain into pleasure—by opening ourselves to deeper connection with ourselves, our partners, and a power beyond ourselves.

As this book progresses you'll find exercises on meditation, giving and receiving, speaking your truth, and connecting with the world around you. To integrate sexuality and spirituality means cultivating love, compassion, and a sense of mystical union—the positive sense of the "Oh God!" feeling. All of these awaken the wisdom and creativity that ancient sages say lie coiled within each of us. In the tradition of Tantric yoga, this energy is called *kundalini* (more about this in chapter 12 on sacred union). Women speak of merging with nature and the elements. They speak of extraordinary light, and visions of "unseen" dimensions. Of moving outside clock time and of traveling effortlessly to "another plane of existence." Of finding that their lives are fuller, richer, and deeper when they return.

As you discover your own paths to sexual desire, may you return with your own stories to tell—beyond the scripts that may have been misinforming you and constricting your sexual development and personal growth. It will become clear as you read on that a major intention of this book is to encourage you to become the author of your own life—to express who you are, what you believe and value, and what you most deeply desire.

4

THE QUEST FOR PARTNERSHIP

I F YOU SPEAK WITH WOMEN away from the roar of medical advice and media hype, if you ask them questions about how sex feels and what it means to them, you'll hear a great many say that the source of their erotic desire is centered in the relationships they have with their partners. Desire doesn't bloom in a lackluster marriage, though. And you don't find Eros hanging around for long among the Bickersons, either—couples who argue with each other in a knock-down struggle for power and control. Ongoing desire and Eros flourish in what wise teachers have called right relationship, where there's a balance of safety and excitement, pleasure and respect, power and nurturing.

True, some of us resist balance. We thrive on adventure and excitement, even yelling matches. We may find that toning ourselves down feels like "mating in captivity," as the title of Esther Perel's thought-provoking book suggests. But by relational balance, I'm not talking about holding back your feelings or trying to overly domesticate each other. I'm talking about practicing fairplay as well as foreplay. What I mean by this is the ability to pay attention to each other's needs as well as your own.

Sexual desire happens in the living room as well as the bedroom. It's connected to our whole lives together. It is nurtured when we talk about our plans, when we make money decisions, and when we do the dishes together. If we don't play fair with one another in these kinds of everyday contexts, desire can go out the window. And I emphasize the *play* aspect of fairplay, too. Sexual desire isn't supposed to be a job of work. It's about feeling good, having fun, and energizing one another.

As you've seen in previous chapters, desire involves many facets of our beings. The flow of desire involves every level of our relationships, too—

from our physical presence to our meetings of heart, mind, and spirit—the urge to reach out beyond ourselves to make contact with each other. Every woman has her own take on which aspects of relationship spark sexual desire, and this holds true whether our partners are men or women—or both. For some of us, it starts with a buff body and physical grace. For others it starts with focused attention and a taste for adventure. One adventurous woman relates that her sexual appetite became "uncontrollable" after her seven-year marriage ended and she began to search for the relationship that was right for her now.

> This sexual desire that was hidden deep finally arose. I felt alive, I wanted to act on all these emotions—so the quest began to find something or someone that would hopefully fulfill all my craving. I tried different avenues of sex from sex toys, boy-toys, movies, bondage, domination, submission, role playing, but nothing or nobody was ever enough. I have such a deep-seated sexual desire that I believe I will never be fulfilled. I'm not looking for Mr. Right—I'm looking for Mr. Sexuality— the man who can take me to that magical place time and time again. If you meet him send him my way.

Other women have a more settled view of sexual desire. A nurse celebrating over two decades of marriage says she believes it flows directly from the life she and her husband have created over the years—the bonding, the trust, the depth of caring and love.

> It's knowing that I can let down my hair and be as free as I want to be with him; knowing that whatever ways we choose to show our love is right for us and brings pleasure to us both in the receiving and in the giving. It is knowing that if the time ever comes that either of us is not capable of physically based love we still have that heart-to-heart, soul-to-soul connection that makes every act we do for one another an act of making love, whether it's a simple kiss or a touch on the cheek, or a

long and lingering caressing look. It is knowing that he is my soulmate, my partner, my best friend, the one who brings joy to my heart and helps me see myself as the woman I want to be, loving, free, part of the Light of the universe.

As this nurse suggests, the kinds of relationships that engender this level of desire are complex. They involve personal self-esteem, loving interaction, and sexual openness. They involve something larger, too—the ability to move beyond the societal conditioning that tells us "good girls don't" and "real men score"—the two-way dynamic I've seen destroy desire for countless couples.

A generous mentor over the years in helping me sort through these relational and societal complexities has been Riane Eisler, a cultural historian and author of many books on the structure of relationships. Her best-known work is *The Chalice and the Blade,* and the one I love best is *Sacred Pleasure,* which charts our history of sex and spirit from cave people to the present day. In both of these books she lays out her partnership model of relationship. I've found this model to be of enormous use to women and couples to help them understand the underlying causes of their discrepancies of sexual desire. Even more important, it offers them positive examples so that they can easily imagine the kind of relationship they crave.

The Partnership Model of Sexual Relationship

Eisler's vision goes galaxies beyond the gender debates that polarize men and women. It also flies beyond the cultural habit of parsing our sexual relationships according to marital status, sexual orientation, or performance—and beyond the medical definitions of sexual health as intercourse with a goal of physical fireworks. She categorizes relationship differences through two constellations of characteristics she identifies as organizing forces in both personal and social contexts. She labels these constellations "dominator" and "partnership" principles of relationship.

DOMINATOR AND PARTNERSHIP MODELS OF SEXUAL RELATIONSHIP

	DOMINATOR MODEL	PARTNERSHIP MODEL
SOCIAL STRUCTURE	Authoritarian	Egalitarian
GENDER RELATIONS	Men outrank women	Gender equality
POWER	Ability to possess and destroy	Ability to love and nurture
CONFLICT RESOLUTION	Decisions by superiors	Attention to mutual wishes and needs
SELF-ESTEEM	Wealth, status, appearance	Emotional and spiritual wishes
PAIR-BONDING	Ownership	Caring
PLEASURE	Suffering is sacred	Joy is sacred
SEXUALITY	Coercion, repression, incest, violence, eroticizing of male dominance	Mutual respect, pleasure, connection, freedom of choice
SPIRITUALITY	Exploitive, punitive divinities	empathic, loving divinities

Adapted from Riane Eisler, *Sacred Pleasure: Sex, Myth, and the Politics of the Body* (San Francisco: HarperCollins, 1995), 403–5.

It's a natural leap to think about Eisler's model in terms of the kinds of sexual relationships that affect our sexual desire. Sexual dominator principles are typified by authoritarian control and lack of empathy—the kind of relationship that can devastate sexual desire for women. Sexual partnership principles are typified by equality and empathic feeling—the kind of relationship so many women say opens them up to sexual pleasure. Let's have a look at what happens with both kinds of relationships.

THE DESIRE TO DOMINATE
"WHY DOESN'T MY WIFE WANT SEX?"

It's easy to visualize dominator principles when you think about Taliban militants or Nazi storm troopers. But there are subtler examples of dominator behavior much closer to home and bedroom—in couples who say they love each other as well as those who are openly hostile. Interestingly, in my experience the first cry for help is often made by a man—who isn't getting what he wants. He comes into my therapy office complaining that his wife or girlfriend isn't interested in sex—and what's the matter with her, anyway?

Let me offer a few speculations, based on stories of hundreds of dominator couples I've worked with over the years. What's the matter with her desire may be that somewhere along the line she has learned to hate herself, and her low self-image results in low sexual desire. What's the matter with her desire may be that he has learned never to be vulnerable and has no clue how to express tenderness and caring, so all she experiences is his constant demand for intercourse—this is increasingly common in this age of Viagra and other pharmaceuticals, because all he has to do is pop a pill and his penis can now perform forever. What's the matter with her desire may be that even though both of them may sincerely want to reach out to each other in love and lust, they're not available to each other because they're each spinning in their own orbits of need or shame or lack of information.

I don't blurt out all these possible scenarios in the first session, not directly anyway. I listen to their stories, which are always unique and rich with detail. But these scenarios are not so far off the national norm. Too many men say women aren't interested. And too many women say their male partners are clueless or bullies, or both. However you slice it, dominator sex almost always results in some kind of desire problem for women, even when it doesn't involve outright cruelty and abuse.

Although sexual desire problems are advertised as a national epidemic, I believe the real epidemic is the dominator dynamic that drains away women's desire. My experience is that dominator couples tend to be low-desire couples because they may not be fully aware of what they're feeling or what's motivating them to be in relationship with one another. Instead of being present for themselves and each other, they may be acting on their ideas of what sex—and each other—are supposed to be.

CULTURAL MISSIONARY POSITION

When women talk about their desire problems, they often frame them as gender complaints. "Most men could care less about women," says one.

"My ex-husband knew only one position and had no clue what a clitoris was," says another. Sometimes I hear women offer grudging compliments followed by a wish for something more: "I finally fell in love with a man who didn't believe that sex is just thrusting and coming for him—but there's still something missing between us."

I've learned that grouchy comments about men usually arise from a complex and troubled history. For many women, dominator dynamics begin early in their lives, with experiences of control, violence, and betrayal—usually (but not always) by men. I've seen it so often I have given it a name. I call it "cultural missionary position"—usually man on top. This is not to slam all men and certainly not to single out your particular father or husband or boyfriend. It is a phrase that simply reflects what I see. And the truth is, men benefit more from the kinds of dominator dynamics Eisler enumerates than women do. So men tend to be less motivated than women to set about changing them.

One of the respondents of my ISIS survey recounts sexual abuse by her stepfather, an uncle, and numerous boyfriends. Her earliest memories include the nightly thuds of her father bashing her mother against the bedroom wall—a routine she now realizes was their prelude to intercourse (she calls it rape). Here's how she says those early experiences impacted her sexual relationships as an adult.

> Since I didn't know any better, I married a similar type of man who only "raped" me once, but beat me senseless with his tongue for over thirty years. And I thought I deserved it. In 1983, when I connected with a women's center and began to learn I had rights, I began to plot my breakaway.

She managed to escape the tongue-lashing husband, but not the dynamic of abuse and put-downs. These stayed with her, and they continue to sap her capacity for sexual desire. Notice that her comments about herself are harsh—as if she's developed a dominator relationship with herself.

> I have an unhealthy attitude about abandonment and rejection. I am very uncomfortable with feeling loved and accepted,

as though I'm not worthy. I'm constantly testing men. I don't believe them or if I do, I'm sure one day, when I'm not aware, they'll turn on me or disappear or do something bad to me. I don't even trust myself. That's sad. But awareness is the first step.

Sexual domination of women is not a new phenomenon of course—and I believe it has always inhibited women's sexual response, especially desire. For our Victorian foremothers, low desire was called "frigidity." Revisionist research now reveals that by no means all Victorian women were ice maidens, but it's easy to guess why some may not have been steamy with lust. Among other inhibitors, they were laced into corsets that prevented their moving freely, let alone taking a full breath.

We never began to learn what was actually happening in American bedrooms until the mid-twentieth century, when sex researcher Alfred Kinsey began his massive surveys on male and female sexual behavior. He never asked a question about abuse or violence. But he did make a startling discovery that may account for low desire on a wide scale. He found that the average amount of time an American couple spent on each incident of intercourse was a mere two minutes. That's less time than it takes me to blow-dry my hair. But apparently it's time enough for Joe Average to mount, ejaculate, and dismount. Granted, Kinsey gathered his data some sixty years ago. But so far nobody's done research that disputes this two-minute figure.

Although the history of sexual desire is rife with stories of cultural missionary position, there is also hope. And as the woman quoted above points out, awareness is the first step.

Of all my client couples who found their paths to sexual awareness, I love the example of the chagrined wife who cried out during her first session with me, "My husband rubs my clitoris as if he's Simonizing his car!" I am not making this up. This couple had sought help for her low sexual desire—and I quickly saw that their issue was more about their dominator conditioning than about her sexual dysfunction. The counseling, of course, had to involve both of them.

I began by explaining the concept of the ISIS Wheel as a way for them to see that there were multiple areas of their relationship that affected their sexual desire. The process helped give them language to organize their thoughts and feelings in a way that didn't cast blame on either of them.

First on the agenda was helping her demonstrate to him that she was a live, pulsing being of flesh and feeling and movement. A close second on the agenda was helping him sensitize his hands to notice that her body had various warm soft places—not chrome headlights that needed to be buffed to a high shine. I suggested he start with her feet, getting to know each toe and heel—then seeing how many other secrets of her body he could discover before working his way back to her clitoris. This exploration moved him to embark on his own ISIS Wheel journey of discovery. He started in the place of emotions to revisit his boyhood messages that guys don't have feelings, they fix things. Both husband and wife were good-humored, eager to learn, and whizzes at their homework, so counseling turned out to be a win-win situation for them. As they developed more sensual flow in their lovemaking and their overall relationship, she became eager for his touch, which now seemed to be soft and responsive.

THE DESIRE FOR PARTNERSHIP
"WE CAN'T KEEP OUR HANDS OFF EACH OTHER."

In contrast to dominator principles, partnership principles are typified by mutual give and take. In terms of sexual desire, this means you notice each other and pay attention to what makes both of you happy. It means you talk together, honestly, about all aspects of your relationship, including the sexual part. It means you put into practice the notion of *fairplay* I introduced at the beginning of this chapter.

I often notice partnership values reflected by the women who come to my workshops—when they talk about the aspects of their sexual stories that they want to keep and build on. They speak of sharing, caring, safety, and pleasure as deep wellsprings of sexual desire. And they underscore the idea that when sexual union is based on partnership values it's likely to be long-lasting because both partners are flexible enough to bend with shifting circumstances over the years: sickness, health, richer, poorer, and so on.

This isn't to say that sexual desire is guaranteed to remain at fever pitch forever if only you care deeply enough about each other and keep fluid lines of communication. It does mean that caring partnerships can weather some of the inevitable relationship shifts, and shifts in sexual desire that occur over the years—though sometimes it seems as if a good thing just seems to keep on keeping on. A sixty-six-year-old retiree writes of her amazement that sex "has only become better with time."

> We can't keep our hands off each other. Any discussion we have invariably means sitting so that we can touch. We agree that whatever has kept us together and loving is not completely understandable, but we're not about to change this good thing that we have.

More than four in five women who responded to my ISIS survey say that the greatest sexual turn-on for them is love. Of course love can mean different things to different people—but the general feeling they convey is one of openness, expansion, trust, and caring. These women also say love connects them with the spirituality of sexual desire—a dynamic we'll visit in more depth in the final chapters of this book.

The retiree above continues her story by saying that for her, desire is embedded in the spiritual and emotional aspects of her relationship, and not in trying to measure up to impossible standards of youth, looks, and agility.

> I believe that in some way our souls have connected in a manner that we are at a loss to explain. I know that when we make love, there is a spiritual joining that enhances the sex. I'm not the most beautiful woman ever and he is not the most handsome man in the world. But, I'm his woman and he's my man. Our love is solid and complete and our sex life is like no other.

Clearly, this woman has moved beyond any stereotypical criteria for a hot, throbbing cycle of desire, arousal, and orgasm. Perhaps this is why she feels she can't find adequate words to explain the erotic quality of the connection with her husband. To her credit, I've found it's often easier to describe the details of dominator sex ("he raped me") than it is to describe the subtle energies that draw us together and inform our lives and partnerships with safety, nurturance, and pleasure. Hopefully a picture of sexual partnership will emerge for you as you continue to read so that you'll be better able to articulate what you want more of in your own life.

Nurturing Sexual Desire in Relationship

Most of our sexual relationships lie on a continuum somewhere between the wholly dominator and the wholly partnership models. Learning to shift your patterns toward partnership can free your flow of desire. Here are some strategies that have worked for women in my practice.

SHARE YOUR FEELINGS WITH YOUR PARTNER
MAKING SPACE FOR DESIRE

Nearly nine out of ten women who answered my ISIS survey say that what makes sex satisfying is sharing deep feelings with their partners—clearly this is consistent with the partnership model of sexual relationship. The kind of sharing this entails is allowing yourself to open up to honest exchanges about what you want, what you don't want, and what your experience means to you. It may mean reminiscing about times you flowed together and sex was effortless and ecstatic. It may mean dredging up pockets of old fear and resentment—the psychic goo we all collect and often seal over for decades, because who wants to revisit all *that* again?

Sharing your deep feelings may mean exploring sexual fantasies together. Your fantasies may be as basic as wishing your partner would hold you and rock you like a baby. Or they may signal your wishes for kinky activities that seem light-years off the normality charts. Sharing any of these feelings and fantasies can be scary, because it brings up the possibility that your partner will ignore you or laugh at you or tell you that what you want is absurd, or even evil—as reported by many women who grew up in Bible Belt, fundamentalist families. But this kind of sharing can be deeply freeing if you can listen to one another without sitting in moral judgment—or mortal terror.

Not all women find it easy to talk about sex, so if "intimacy interruptus" is a predicament that's familiar in your life, you have plenty of company. Many women find that the luxury of sexual play becomes subsumed in the busyness of their lives. After the first flush of falling in love, you may need to create regular occasions to be alone together if you want to keep exercising your capacity for deep sexual intimacy. The attempt to make protected time can bring into sharp focus just how many anti-intimacy tactics you may employ—or that may employ you. Raise your hand if you recognize any of these: TV, cell phone, e-mail, kids, dogs, shopping, sleep, your exercise program, your hair, your blog, your job . . .

But it's crucial to understand that sexual communication is much more than just making intimacy dates. And it clearly involves more than two-minute intercourse. True sexual sharing is an ongoing happening. It radiates throughout your body, your breath, your smile, your smell, your dress, your attitude, your hair follicles, your whole being—in the bedroom and beyond. An energized colleague points out that she and her husband can communicate volumes simply by gazing into each other's eyes—even after four years of marriage, and even in a crowded lunch place: "It's as much making love—and as satisfying—as when we're in bed together."

You might find it helpful to begin by hearing how other women feel about sex and what it means to them. There are some wonderful books on sexual communication in the Suggested Readings at the end of this book—and some wonderful first-person stories in my previous book *The Heart and Soul of Sex,* which is based on survey responses of thousands of women. But all the reading in the world can't replace the kinds of understanding that grows with the partnership qualities we can develop together through opening ourselves to pleasure—and taking the risk of letting each other know about it.

Invite each other to share a new level of partnership
A vow of friendship

In the summer of 1999, I was in the throes of analyzing my ISIS survey results, and totally ready to shake off all the academic dust I'd collected. I leapt at the chance to camp out with a group of healers and environmentalists on retreat in the wilds of northern Vermont. The place was called Far Out Field not only because it was light-years away from the nearest fast-food chain, but also because it was vast and commanded magical views of sunrise and moonrise over the Green Mountains. The first morning I woke to find tucked into my tent flap a small card that held a big message:

Druid Vow of Friendship

I honor your gods
I drink from your well
I bring an unprotected heart to our meeting place
I will not negotiate by withholding
I hold no cherished outcome
I am not subject to disappointment

These simple lines were extraordinarily moving to me at the time, and they continue to move me years later as I write this chapter. I've kept this saying taped to my office wall and have used it as inspiration and guidance for myself and others.

This vow epitomizes all of the partnership principles outlined earlier. It also taps into the hunger for relationships that involve body, mind, heart, and spirit. It works for more than just friendships, too. Over the years, I've given copies of this vow to couples who come to me seeking deeper understanding with one another. And I've handed it to women in my workshops—letting them parse its meaning for themselves. Here, let's explore its message line by line, and see what it can tell us about creating—and maintaining—a true partnership flow of sexual desire. But don't take my word for it. See what it can mean for you.

I honor your gods. When you begin a relationship, you bring with you all the traditions and beliefs you've developed before you ever met. These range from spiritual and religious customs to attitudes about love and making love. Loving well takes much more than merely tolerating each other's beliefs. To fully "honor each other's gods" acknowledges deep respect for all that your partner holds dear—even when that differs from some of what you hold dear. What does this have to do with sexual desire? Women say that this kind of loving respect allows for connection at the very deepest level of trust. And it's not only women who believe this. It was Fritz Perls, the founder of Gestalt therapy, who famously said, "Contact is the appreciation of differences."

I drink from your well. I take this sentence as a classic statement of caring for one another's physical well-being. In early societies drinking from a neighbor's well meant receiving a gift of the water necessary for sustaining life. In terms of sexual relationship, what this conveys to me is a sense of safety—that sense of "coming home" so many couples describe when they speak of curling into each other's bodies at night—as if that contact is a deep well of pleasure to which each has open access.

I bring an unprotected heart to our meeting place. Openheartedness is essential for the care and feeding of sexual desire. How can we love each other if our hearts are so bound up in protective armor that we can't feel? Letting go of defenses, sharing our feelings, empathic listening, and touching each other's hearts are all part of filling the deep longings for sexual connection. It's what women mean when they say: "We don't just have sex—we make love."

I will not negotiate by withholding. Over history, women have been the sexual gatekeepers. Withholding sex is one way we've been able to live up to the injunction "good girls don't." It's also how we've been able to assert some measure of power and control over dominator partners who want to keep us in perpetual cultural missionary position—barefoot, pregnant, and doing all the housework. In partnership relationships we have the opportunity to rethink our position. We can be "good" and still desire sexual pleasure, orgasm, and ecstasy. And we have the permission and the power to ask for what we want—whether it's for more clitoral stimulation or for our partners to pick up the kitchen.

I hold no cherished outcome. What a crucial statement this line makes for keeping sexual desire alive. It conveys to me a willingness to be in the present rather than on a relentless quest for sexual goals—intercourse, multiple orgasm, a major "score." Letting go of sexual goals doesn't mean giving up on sex. It means opening up to possibilities that may not have entered your consciousness yet. You may be in for a treat. Women often call this the desire for "something more."

I am not subject to disappointment. In today's post-Viagra world, a dynamic sex life has become an expectation. It's easy to feel grouchy about ourselves and others if we think we're falling short of this ideal. To declare yourself immune to disappointment makes a powerful statement about willingness to take responsibility for your own pleasure. There's an intrinsic optimism here. You can handle whatever unfolds—no matter what others say. You can weather relational storms, past, present, and future. You have the power to be in a place of serenity.

One of the great lessons I take from this view of friendship is that your relationship with your partner boils down to right relationship with yourself. In the next chapter, we'll look at how you can begin to create a self-affirming sense of your own potential as a sexual—and spiritual—being.

5

MÉNAGE À MOI
Creating Partnership with Yourself

ENTER THE DREADED M-WORD. Talking about masturbation isn't easy in this culture, especially for women, because we're not supposed to talk about sex at all—at least not the part where we enjoy it. And certainly not the part where we may enjoy it more with ourselves than we do with our partners. And double-certainly not the part where we glory in the sheer independence and pleasure of our sexual responses whether we have partners or not. The law of the land says that sex is supposed to happen between couples, preferably male and female.

But call it self-pleasure, self-abuse, or *ménage à moi*, masturbation is far more than just a scary word. It can be a surefire route to desire and orgasm, and it's the safest sex going. Touching yourself for pleasure involves all of you—how you think and feel as well as your physical sensations.

To have a sexual experience with yourself, and say so out loud, is one of the most highly charged topics in the sexual lexicon. Sex researcher Martha Cornog, who provided the wonderful phrase *ménage à moi*, tells the whole story of it in her *Big Book of Masturbation*. The very idea of masturbation has created controversy through history and across cultures—since well before St. Augustine officially proclaimed it to be a sin. Masturbation taboos have created a raft of classic myths ("You'll go blind!") and jokes ("Couldn't I just do it till I need to wear glasses?"). Rules to keep us from touching ourselves "down there" have been codified by the most powerful institutions of the Western world—religion, law, and medicine. And let's not forget the media—newspapers, magazines, and television have kept it a dirty secret. But not the Internet, which boasts millions of sites that offer information, encouragements, and of course sleaze when it comes to the subject of masturbation.

Rules against self-pleasure apply to men as well as women. In today's world the rules seem to fall on men a little less harshly, however. After all, boys will be boys, wink, wink. And nice girls—well, nice girls *don't*. More than half the women in the United States still have problems touching themselves, according to a variety of studies. This percentage may or may not be accurate, though. My educated guess is that many more women may feel more comfortable about touching themselves than they do about saying that they do.

It's not surprising that the women's liberation movement in the 1970s flexed its collective muscles to try to lift the taboos off the M-word. Leading the way were books like *Our Bodies, Ourselves* in 1973 and Betty Dodson's subversive pamphlet "Liberating Masturbation" in 1972, which morphed into her best-selling book, *Sex for One*. Many a woman who came of age sexually during those years still remembers the awesome moment of taking a mirror in hand to examine herself "down there." Or taking a vibrator in hand to test the theory that the clitoris is the only organ of the body whose one and only and wonderful purpose is pleasure. *Our Bodies, Ourselves* is still going strong—in 2005 it celebrated its thirty-fifth anniversary with its latest revised edition. Betty Dodson's still going strong, too, in her late seventies, with a provocative new video and a website that rocks: www. BettyDodson.com.

There have been outspoken political voices for masturbation, as well. Three recent U.S. surgeons general—C. Everett Koop, Joycelyn Elders, and David Satcher—have supported it as a method of safe and responsible sexual expression, especially for young people, who are so often at risk for sexually transmitted infections. Dr. Satcher pronounced masturbation to be a public health asset rather than a moral hazard—read his landmark 2001 *Call to Action to Promote Sexual Health and Responsible Sexual Behavior*. Still, the stigma lingers. Dr. Elders was forced to resign as surgeon general on December 1, 1994—a direct outcome of having said "yes" at a World AIDS Day conference when asked if she thought sex education courses should teach that masturbation is a safe alternative to intercourse.

The Do-It-Yourself Model of Sexual Desire

Many women say they prefer to be sexual with a partner rather than with themselves alone. But masturbation has its partnership upside, too. As one woman quipped in the 1976 *Hite Report on Women's Sexuality:* "At least I get to go to bed with someone I like." The problem arises when your self-esteem takes a nosedive. Early in my career as a therapist, a client admitted to me: "But I'm not so sure I like myself."

Like so many women, this woman felt conflicted and guilty—like a bad girl for enjoying how good it felt to touch her own clitoris and breasts. It was as if she had somehow internalized a teensy Nancy Reagan in a red dress wagging her finger and mouthing "Just Say No."

Self-esteem is clearly a primary factor in sexual desire. It starts with right relationship with yourself. When you masturbate, you take the responsibility for sexual pleasure literally into your own hands. In fact, sex therapists routinely prescribe it as "homeplay" for women who need to know more about their sexual responses—what they like, what they don't like, how they feel, how they can be independently sexual, and how they can gather crucial clues for their sexual partners.

The truth is, sexual desire doesn't always involve an intimate *other.* Sex educators and scientists emphasize that we're sexual beings throughout our lives—and there's no way any of us can have access to a sexual partner all of that time. Certainly not when we're children, possibly not in our later years, and probably not every one of the years in between—think sporadic dating, think celibacy, think divorce, think death of a partner.

So without a partner, how are you as a sexual being supposed to express your sexuality? The obvious answer is: with the person who knows you best; the most dependable sexual partner you'll ever have; the partner who's guaranteed never to leave until death do you part. News flash! That's *you.*

Exploring Your Sexual Desire
Using the ISIS Model to Affirm Your Self

Back to my client who'd internalized the big red "no" message about self-pleasure. Clearly this woman had work to do. But we soon discovered that the work wasn't all about her flagging self-esteem. It was also about broadening her perspective on masturbation. She needed to learn how the negative messages she'd absorbed from girlhood on had all conspired to short circuit her sexual desire. She needed to learn that her negative responses were perfectly normal—if "normal" means that most women feel that way.

Our first step was to help her find some "yes" messages. We began by using the template of the ISIS Wheel in chapter 1 to illustrate that erotic touching isn't limited to just the physical part of yourself. It's part of the whole pattern of desire. That is, it's also possible to touch yourself emotionally, mentally, and spiritually. This template helped give her a comprehensive perspective so that she could locate which of her paths of desire were open and which ones were blocked.

The physical path was a natural place for my client to start because she could easily identify the sensations. She also found herself able to experience the emotional path—because she felt so joyous about finally allowing herself to say "yes" from her heart. The mental and spiritual paths were more difficult for her, because she was still fighting that old "no" voice that told her touching herself was immoral, disgusting, and evil. Ultimately, soul-talks with several of her woman friends helped free her from the fear that she was the only one who felt twirled by all her conflicting feelings.

What I've learned from working with countless clients and also from my own life is that pleasuring yourself can be a crucial part of the journey of self-awareness. You move along at your own pace. And it doesn't have to be a lonely trek beset by wrathful deities. It can be a journey of personal wholeness, for pleasuring yourself involves much more than your body. You're involving your mind, emotions, and spirit too. When your involvement is strong, you can forge a sense of sexual partnership with yourself. Some women experience this process as a sacred union—of their male and female aspects. Some feel it as a bringing together of other so-called dualities, such as body and spirit, giver and receiver, survivor and healer. In this sense, it can become a relational journey as well—even when you're alone. And any sex therapist will tell you that masturbating with a partner is a fabulous way of demonstrating exactly where and how you like to be touched.

I love the story told by a fifty-six-year-old Hawaii artist because it illustrates so many of these aspects of self-pleasure. The kind of information she offers is extraordinary—and so therapeutic I wish she'd been around to help counsel the client above. This artist describes how a "routine bedtime meditation" evolved into an ecstatic sexual experience for her—and how that ecstasy elicited an ongoing spiritual quest. One of the impressive aspects of her story is that she didn't enter into her masturbation experience as a accomplished pro. Like so many women who've been told "don't touch yourself down there," she entered tentatively, and then found herself gradually opening up and letting go.

> I began to experience a very sensual, sexual flow, buildup, then an all-pervading rush of energy. At the time, I'd not heard of *kundalini,* or anything of that nature. Shortly, I had an overwhelming experience of transcendence and Oneness with the Divine as I understood it at the time.

Her reference to *kundalini* comes from Tantric yoga. According to this ancient system, the body's sexual energy flows upward from the base of the spine to the crown of the head. An open flow allows for the union of female and male energies—the goddess Shakti meets the god Shiva. The result is sacred partnership with one's self. And this is exactly what this woman describes—in her own terms.

> I realized in a moment that seemed to last an eternity, that I was experiencing a sexual union of my body/mind/spirit with the All-and-the-Everything, with God and Goddess altogether as One, as my Self. I was experiencing some kind of ecstatic orgasm, for lack of a better description. It took over completely and literally "blew my mind" and everything else of my personal self. I was alone in my home at the time. I recall too that as I was undergoing this experience, a strong gust of wind came up and blew forcefully through the rooms of the house! When the orgasmic experience was over, I lay on the carpeted floor, panting for breath, then very still. I was filled with "the peace that passeth all understanding."

The return from her journey was far from peaceful though. She describes it as confusing and painful—for she had to re-enter daily life where gods and goddesses don't exist and where connecting sex and spirit is still taboo, along with masturbation. She experienced classic symptoms of psychic culture shock. She was disoriented and weepy, and afraid to talk about her experience.

> As I gathered myself together and got up off the floor to get ready for bed, I realized that I also felt embarrassed. Then, surprisingly, I felt a deep grief, an abysmal loss, of something extremely sacred that I could not even name. I recall that I stayed in a state of lethargy and mourning for about two days following that experience.

When she emerged from mourning, she resolved to get to know the male and female aspects of herself—her internal meeting of Shakti and Shiva. In the process, she entered into what she calls a "covenant" with herself—a sacred union that went well beyond the Mars and Venus model of relationship we're taught is the norm in this culture.

As so many other women have related to me, she found that her solo experience profoundly influenced other aspects of her life. She writes that she's now less prone to judging others or trying to control them. Having so fully experienced that most intimate of sexual partnerships—with herself—she says she's able to reach out more confidently and compassionately into the world around her. And a surprise benefit: She says her new and larger concept of self has vastly enriched her sexual relationship with her husband.

The Art of Self-Pleasure
Discovering Your Own Gifts

When you learn the art of self-pleasure, you begin to discover special gifts of sexual desire. There is the self-acceptance and openness that come with getting to know yourself sexually. There's the serenity that comes with trusting that you can anticipate a safe and entertaining evening with yourself instead of feeling lonely and unloved. There's the willingness to take charge of your own sexual pleasure and the freedom you give yourself to be a delicious lover without involving a sexual partner other than your-self. Along the way you may have to cope with the fear of breaking the rules that say you're supposed to depend on a man to fulfill your sexual needs. (Or was that fulfill *his* sexual needs?) And you may have to deal with pernicious guilt—especially religious guilt—for whatever the female equivalent is of the biblical Onan "spilling his seed upon the ground." And God forbid you should take time just for yourself. Just for sexual pleasure. Aren't you supposed to be doing something worthwhile with your time? Knitting socks for the troops, maybe.

Most of all, the art of self-pleasure involves listening closely to your-self—whether you make an extended appointment with yourself or are enjoying a quickie. What patterns and rituals awaken your senses and sen-sibilities? Where do you like to touch yourself? And how? How do you breathe? How do you move your body? What's going through your mind? Do you like to make sounds? What happens to your energy as you pleasure yourself? Some women can feel themselves light up. Their pelvises glow, their hearts and throats open, their whole bodies pulse and hum. What does the aftermath feel like? What do you carry with you as you continue on with your day? What do you carry into your dreams at night?

Maybe you simply dive in, letting your lust or the memory of other times carry you along the pleasure path. But some women need props and prepa-ration for erotic pleasure. Perhaps a glass of wine or spring water. Perhaps a favorite sexual fantasy. Perhaps setting the scene with flowers, music, candles, and incense. Some women start with prayer and meditation. For others, self-pleasuring involves luxurious bathing—dripping water, sen-suous steam, scented oils, playful exploration of the body.

With a little imagination you can turn your tub or shower into a spa or leafy tropical paradise. The water from faucet or showerhead can become the liquid lover you always dreamed of, and you can orchestrate the experi-ence yourself. The point is, there are many ways to enjoy sensual, sexual pleasure without a partner. Or to pleasure yourself even when you're with a partner.

At the risk of taxing your belief system, I want to point out the intrinsic divinity of the sexy activities listed above. All of them have their roots in religious ritual. It's true. In early cultures, sexual pleasure was included in the worship of all things, and vestiges of sexual activities remain in our religious rituals today, though they're well purged of any intention for sexual pleasure. Think about what happens in your house of worship. Is there laying on of hands? Anointing with oil? Immersion in water? Setting the scene with flowers, incense, candles, music, and wine? I could go on. We'll talk more about this in chapter 12, on sacred union.

I don't claim this radical idea as my own. I first encountered it in my conversations with Riane Eisler, who was joining Marija Gimbutas and other feminist anthropologists in asking new questions about ancient myths and artifacts: How come so many early creation stories begin with sexual union? Why does this Sumerian Artemis figure have so many breasts? And oh, look—in that Paleolithic cave painting in Lascaux, France, the hand of the Mother Goddess is pointing to her genitals.

So, counterintuitive though it might sound, engaging in rituals of self-pleasure may be connecting you directly with your spiritual goddess roots whether or not you're aware this is happening. And clearly, these rituals can be a way into your personal ISIS Wheel, connecting your sensations, thoughts, and feelings about sexual experience. Either way, remember the Hawaii artist above. Self-pleasure can take you to far places. So be prepared to experience energetic shifts that may go well beyond orgasm and even beyond physical sensation.

The Hand or the Vibrator?

What about vibrators and other sex toys? Many women prefer their hands, and some see vibrators as mechanical intrusions onto the natural scene. But when push comes to shove, no human hand can match the tireless stimulation of an electric vibrator, and there are women who need this amount of direct stimulation to bring themselves to orgasm. As a friend remarked recently, when pleasure's on the line, it's important to call in all your allies.

How do you choose a vibrator? The varieties are seemingly endless, and almost all in designer colors. Besides plug-ins, you can get battery-operated ones. There are even vibrators than function under water. You can accessorize them to ramp up pleasure for every inch of your genitalia—clitoris, labia, G-spot, you name it.

A caveat on cordless models. Make sure you remove any batteries prior to air travel. A colleague was involved in a most embarrassing incident when the switch of her lavender silicone "Lickin' Lizard" flipped on inside her suitcase during an airport inspection. Officials ripped her baggage apart, held her rotating reptile aloft, and guffawed lewdly. She was lucky she wasn't detained as a threat to national security.

Can you become addicted to your vibrator? This is a subject for debate among aficionadas, and a question only you can answer for yourself. True addiction is a serious personality disorder. But if you're concerned about becoming too dependent on your vibrator, ask yourself if what you're really worried about is wanting too much pleasure—such a taboo for women. Or maybe your partner's nose is out of joint because you're having phenomenal orgasmic experiences all by yourself. In this case, why not introduce your partner to your vibrator and enjoy some threesome pleasure?

More than one client has confided to me that she considers her vibrator to be her significant other. Which is fine if you don't have a partner. But if you find that your vibrator use is really getting between you and your flesh-and-blood partner, take it seriously. Talk with yourself. Talk with your partner. Talk with your vibrator even. If these conversations don't change things, there's help available—see the Resources section at the end of this book for counseling suggestions.

Even beyond the closed doors of the bedroom, plenty of controversy swirls about vibrators. Read Rachel Maines's eye-opening book, *The Technology of Orgasm*, which details how physicians once used an astonishing array of mechanical vibrators to bring their female patients to orgasm. I am not making this up. Before current codes of medical ethics, periodic masturbation by a physician was a standard treatment to calm the recurring symptoms of "hysteria"—known for centuries as "wandering womb." And did you know there's a law on the books in Texas that says you can go to jail for owning more than six vibrators. Six? Suppose you have a partner—can you own twelve between you? See the delightful film *Passion and Power*, based on Maines's book and produced by Wendy Slick and Emiko Omori, which shows and tells the story. At its 2007 premiere to an audience of sexuality educators and therapists, this documentary received an extended standing O.

A good (and safe) place to learn about vibrators and other sex toys is through women's sexuality boutiques. Yes, these exist, and they're very different from the "adult" sex shops in your local red light district. The Resources section lists several innovative women-owned sexuality boutiques along with their websites. Eve's Garden in New York City and Good Vibrations in San Francisco are the ones I know best. The founders are sex-educator colleagues, and their emphasis is on safety and empowerment as well as fun. If you're able to visit their stores, you'll meet creative salespeople who can help you decide if vibrators or other sex toys are for you. If you can't get to a store personally, their websites are an education in themselves.

Where's the spirituality factor in vibrator use? Freedom! A sexy-though-single teacher describes her twelve celibate years as a divorcée, during which she discovered that she was free at last—and that sex could fill her spiritual longings as well as her physical ones.

> I threw off the old no-nos of "ugly body," "girls don't enjoy sex," "never sleep with a man you aren't married to." I discovered through masturbation that I liked sex! It was fun! Girls could enjoy it! I got a vibrator and learned to use it. I watched some X-rated films to learn what gave me pleasure and I learned to pleasure myself.

Controversy swirls about "X-rated films," too, and with good cause. The pornography industry is infamously exploitive of women. Moreover, it promotes limited (and often violent) views of sex—it's the dominator model in living color. But because so much information about sex is suppressed in this culture, these films fill an inimitable role in sex education. They represent one of the few ways we can actually see explicit sexual activities—so that, as the woman above explains, we can learn what gives us pleasure and what turns us off.

There are explicit films that show a wider range of sexual activities than down and dirty porn, and that tend to be more sensitive to what women want. They also tend to focus on relationships as a way of building desire, and may incorporate a bit of humor, too. Check out Candida Royalle's

Femme Productions, the first woman-run erotic film company. Also check out the explicit educational films that feature sex-therapist commentary on sexual activities, such as the highly advertised "Better Sex" series by Sinclair Films. If sacred sexuality and Tantra interest you, there are growing numbers of sensuous and instructive films. For some women, like the teacher above, watching films like these helps them lay to rest some old bugaboos and take charge of their own sexual story.

I cannot end this chapter without mentioning the online sexual worlds that exist—beyond just looking at photos or watching movies. In recent years, more interactive modes of cybersex have emerged, and these have millions of devotees—mostly twenty-somethings I imagine. Here, you can create your own sexual reality in the form of "avatars"—cyber characters who can do on your computer whatever you've always wanted to do in the flesh. Nothing is off-limits—you can mix gender, race, even species. You can "marry" other avatars or spirit them off to nether regions. Says Todd Melby, senior writer for the AASECT monthly journal *Contemporary Sexuality*, the 3-D virtual world of Second Life (www.secondlife.com) is a place you can bring your real-life attitudes or try out new ones. "You are responsible for creating the kind of world you want to live in. You're also responsible for creating the kind of person (or mammal or dragon or whatever) you want to be."

Whether or not you decide to create a virtual "second life" as part of your personal ménage à moi, I encourage you to keep a record of your own story. Put a journal by your bed. Jot down your journey as you discover your special paths of pleasure and self-pleasure. Notice what comes up for you physically, mentally, emotionally, and spiritually. This is a practical and simple way you can follow your ISIS Wheel experiences. And you may find that recording your experiences gives them special meaning for you.

In the next section we'll look at a number of specific problems that can act as roadblocks to desire—and see that the ISIS Wheel offers to expand your sexual desire by opening your consciousness, with yourself and with your partner. If you're concerned about changes you feel you may have to make, take a deep breath and relax. The changes may not be so very huge. Maybe just a shift in your intention, suggests research psychoanalyst Paul Joannides in his *Guide to Getting It On*. He points out that even small shifts can lead to wide openings in experience. For instance, when a surfer leads with the right foot instead of the left, it can result in a totally different experience of the wave. So think of desire as a wave. Perhaps if you begin approaching it in a different way, your whole experience will shift.

Part Two

∞

Why WOMEN SAY NO *to* SEX

And How to Find Your Way Back to Yes

REFLECTIONS

What's made you say no? What's helped you say yes?

Sex was just depressing with my husband of twenty years. During my separation I began nurturing myself for the first time. And loving myself. By getting "healthy" I attracted a healthier man who adores all of me.

    —Forty-five-year-old business owner from Colorado Springs, Colorado

When I finally broke out of the trap of my childhood religious training, when I realized that repressing sexuality repressed love, peace, and oneness, among other things, I finally let go of the guilt and began to enjoy sex.

    —Thirty-eight-year-old stockbroker from New Orleans, Louisiana

Having been sexually abused as a child has *hugely* affected my sexuality although it is not always clear how. I am trying to slowly let go of the belief that my sexuality is bad or shameful. Sexual intimacy is one thing that heals those wounds.

    —Twenty-six-year-old actor from Norfolk, Virginia

Loving someone that loves you back makes all the difference. Being with a woman was a big eye-opener for me. For the first time in my life I made a love/spiritual connection.

    —Twenty-seven-year-old social worker from St. Paul, Minnesota

I have been without a partner since his stroke, five years ago. I am fifty-five and I have learned to satisfy myself. Who needs a man? It's not in the other person but in yourself!

    —Fifty-five-year-old sales manager from Phoenix, Arizona

6

LOSING YOURSELF IN YOUR PARTNER
When Relationships That Seem Made in Heaven
Turn Out to Be from Hell

AS WE'VE SEEN THROUGHOUT PREVIOUS CHAPTERS, broadening our notion of sexual desire can open us to deeper pleasures and more meaningful partnerships. But the paths of life and love are seldom smooth. The bumpy ride may begin with exchanges around money and housework. Then we have babies, or engage in affairs, or fall in love with another woman, or find ourselves face to face with memories of early abuse. Any of these can cause our sexual responses to go haywire—which may lead us to believe there's something wrong with us on top of everything else. Therapist's offices are filled with women wringing their handkerchiefs because they fear they've failed at sex.

In this section we'll look at all of these issues and suggest how you can use the ISIS Wheel to bring sexual balance and vibrancy back into your life. Let's start with one of the most common desire slayers I hear women report: sexual codependency—a continual pattern of focusing on your partner's needs until you lose your sense of self. Too many of us have been taught this is how we're supposed to attract our partners and keep them interested. But when we abandon our own identity—poof! there goes sexual desire. A disillusioned client voiced the problem in compelling terms: "One day I went to look for myself and there was no one there."

In my practice over the years I've seen countless women who have lost themselves in their sexual partners. It's as if they moved in to the relationship with all their emotional furniture, and can't find their way back home again. They end up living their partners' lives instead of their own. Their confidence plummets; they feel unsafe, uncared for, and unable to nurture themselves. Their operative phrase is: "Without you I am nothing."

In this place of "nothing" there's little room for a smooth flow of sexual desire. Desire may slow to a trickle, caught in a morass of low self-worth and impossible fantasies. Or it may gush forth in ways that invite disappointment, rejection, even violence. What started out as your honeymoon dream may end up a nightmare over the long term. And sexual desire is one of the things that go bump in the night.

The desire for sexual closeness is part of the natural process of bonding and attachment. The longing to reach into each other's core can run deep. For many lovers, heart-to-heart connection is life-sustaining and expanding—as if you and your partner are each other's personal portals into the eternal mysteries. This is especially true when you're in the raptures of new love. You are nectar to one another. You live for each other's energy. "We feed each other spiritually and emotionally," says a colleague of her relationship with her new "soulmate."

Although sexual connection can be a wellspring of creativity and hope and delight, there can be a sinister side, too. I've met self-described love junkies—men as well as women—who use it the way substance abusers use drugs and alcohol. They can't ever get enough, and nobody can ever fill their needs. Some try to recreate the sexual high by falling in love over and over again, without regard for the lovers they may leave strewn by the wayside.

Love can get "old" in a hurry, when you're one of the ones who's being strewn—though if your self-esteem is at low enough tide, you may put up with outrageous behavior long past the time it serves either of you. I know this dynamic well. In my thirties I went through five soul-punishing years with a man who abandoned me every evening—the minute he had his first drink. Though he wasn't throwing me aside for another woman, he staged continual disappearing acts that sometimes turned downright mean. Toward the end there wasn't much positive energy left between us, but I couldn't let go. I was terrified he'd leave for real and I'd have to figure out life on my own. I remember sobbing on a friend's shoulder and actually uttering the classic words, "BUT I LOVE HIM!" My friend's response helped change the course of that marriage—and my life. "Gina," she said without a shred of humor, "that's not love; that's something you talk to a shrink about."

Now, long years later (and trained to be the kind of "shrink" other lovelorn women talk to), I think I've finally learned to differentiate between love and need. Love comes from a fully filled personal well and is about opening up your heart to others. Need comes from an empty personal well and is about seeking approval and nurturing from others—too often from other empty souls who are incapable of intimacy. These are oversimplifications to be sure, but they point up an essential truth: when the desire for closeness is born of emptiness, the result is bound to be constriction, not expansion. The minute you feel "I am nothing without you," closeness shape-shifts into smothering. Flirting turns into hostage taking. Sexual desire morphs into relational quicksand that will suck you down faster than you can cry out, "What is this thing called love?" I've seen clients so subsumed in their partners that they seem to disappear. Journalist Sheila Graham phrased it poignantly back in the 1930s when she wrote to her lover F. Scott Fitzgerald, "If only I could walk into your eyes and pull the lids behind me and leave all the world outside."

Her words epitomize desperate longing for connection and protection—a condition I've witnessed far too many women feeling today. And they stand as warning that the desire to merge totally with your partner can become a dead end—a kind of great escape to Nowheresville. The shorthand label for this situation is "codependency." My colleague Wendy Maltz (*The Sexual Healing Journey*) reminds me that labels are for jelly jars, not for people. Still, I think it helps to have a code word to signify that the insatiable drive to lose yourself in someone else differs from the interdependent give and take of vibrant sexual partnership.

In case you're wondering, sexual codependency is not all about knuckling under to a man. Lesbian women describe falling into it, too. In fact, when both partners in a relationship are women it can be even more difficult to see the interplay of how one partner is absorbed by another. Or how both may be simultaneously absorbed by each other. As one lesbian client put it: "We think alike. We dress alike. It's easy to be dysfunctional alike, too." And sexual desire can suffer, too. We'll have a look at so-called lesbian bed death in chapter 10.

When Sexual Desire Meets Codependency

If merging with our partners starts out feeling so good, how do we get to the place where we're isolated and diminished rather than expanded? How do we know when sexual connection and bonding are out of balance? And what happens to sexual desire?

You know your relationship is out of whack when you feel angst instead of pleasure. You feel stagnancy instead of movement and flow. But mostly you have the eerie sense that what's fueling your sexual desire—or siphoning it away—is not coming entirely from *you*. In my 1990 book *Sexual Recovery*, I define sexual codependency as a painful pattern of lovemaking in which your attitudes and behaviors are habitually determined by someone else—and not by yourself. Inspirational writer Vernon Howard describes codependency more colorfully. He says it feels like letting the waiter eat your dinner. I love this description and quote it often because it so graphically describes the abrupt twirling of high expectations.

With these definitions in mind you can begin to see that what look like women's desire problems aren't always problems with sexual response. The real problem may be that women get so wrapped up in pleasing their partners they neglect themselves. They may knock themselves out to look good, dress seductively, and focus on their partners' wants long beyond the point when these actions hold intrinsic pleasure for them. It's not that these women have too much or too little sexual drive. It's that they no longer want to engage in sexual activity because it's too often resulted in failure, disappointment, and hurt.

Being in this kind of relational quagmire doesn't necessarily mean you're sick or bad or dysfunctional. Above all, it doesn't mean you have to stay trapped there for life. Instead, it may mean that you've taken your "good girl" conditioning to a level that doesn't serve you well in the present. Chances are you're a well-socialized woman, doing exactly what you've been trained to do since you were playing Barbie dress-up—when you learned to take care of everyone else's needs and feelings before you got around to considering your own. But this kind of caretaking can be painful for you. It can be frustrating for your partner, too—who may actually hold your well-being as a priority. And it can kill sexual desire dead— pow, right through the heart. It never had a chance, they said, standing over the inert relationship.

Connectedness and Codependency
Walking the Fine Line

There can be a surprisingly fine line between an ecstatic sense of oneness with your partner and the kind of nuclear fusion that erases your sense of sexual self. From what I've seen, the difference often begins with what each of you brings into the relationship. That means your early experience and training—all those years of reacting to the "thou shalts" and "thou shalt nots" you grew up with, along with any experiences of cruelty or abuse.

Most likely your sexual attitudes were formed in your family. Also in school. Also in your place of religious worship. And what you believe now about sex can depend on the community you grew up in, too. As we've seen in previous chapters, there's a whole range of cultural messages that affect us—and the contemporary community standards of sexual behavior may differ greatly from place to place. A Minnesota camp counselor says she had to shed layers and layers of "Lutheran guilt." A Georgia realtor says she had to move beyond the "hypocrisy, bigotry and dogma in the old town Presbyterian Church." Women from all over the country say they've had to shed the notion that they're supposed to worship the "other"—something or someone outside themselves—as if they're incapable of finding meaning in their own lives.

The truth is, the kind of sexual desire that touches us deeply tends to flourish when we feel safe, self-confident, caring, cared for, powerful, and pleasure-loving. And this is true whether we're eighteen or eighty-six. But when sexual attraction is born out of low self-esteem, fear, neediness, and pain, it may feel as if one partner is doing all the giving and the other is only taking. In fact, both partners may feel as if they're not receiving nearly enough.

ASSESSING YOUR SELF AND YOUR RELATIONSHIP

If you experience a discrepancy in giving and receiving, here's a simple awareness exercise that can help you assess your sense of self in relationship. Some women find this is an important first step toward rebalancing their patterns of sexual desire and satisfaction.

Below are six pairs of opposite feeling states. This is not a "laundry list"—a litany of all-encompassing traits that's designed to show how dysfunctional you are. Rather, this list reflects a range of feelings that all of us experience at one time or another. This is your opportunity to show how they figure in your sexual relationships. The value of this exercise isn't to produce a glowing profile—that's just as counterproductive as memorizing the eye chart when you go for your annual checkup. It's to open discussion between you and your partner so you can assess what underlies your sexual desire—or lack of it.

Check the line segment closest to the statement that best reflects your own experience. Note that there are six line segments so you can't just indicate "I don't know" by checking the middle. There are no right or wrong answers—the idea is to identify what you perceive to be true for you.

WHAT IS YOUR SENSE OF YOURSELF?

Safe	_ _ _ _ _ _	Afraid
Self-confident	_ _ _ _ _ _	Insecure
Nurtured	_ _ _ _ _ _	Needy
Nurturing	_ _ _ _ _ _	Careless
Powerful	_ _ _ _ _ _	Victimized
Pleasure-loving	_ _ _ _ _ _	In pain
Other	_ _ _ _ _ _	Other
Other	_ _ _ _ _ _	Other

Ask your partner to do this exercise as well. Then share your observations. Once you can each clearly identify your sense of safety, self-confidence, and so on, you'll be better able to discuss your feelings together—which can be a next step toward rebalancing sexual desire and satisfaction.

For double awareness, go through this list again with your partner, and rank how you imagine *each other* falls between each of these opposites. You may be surprised. Some couples who think they know each other inside and out end up with an entirely new take on what's really happening in their relationships.

Doing this exercise may be scary or difficult at first. But see if it's an improvement over focusing only on what you imagine might please each other. (When I was on the codependency lecture circuit in the 1980s, the running joke was: "When a codependent dies somebody *else's* life flashes before her eyes.")

Assessing your sexual roles

Another way to assess the quality of sexual connectedness in your relationship is through the lens of your sexual roles. Are you playing roles that bring you into vital sexual connection? Or are you locked into roles that keep you distant from each other? On the next page are some roles inspired by Riane Eisler's dominator-partnership model, which is outlined in chapter 4. Roles that enhance positive sexual partnership are likely to lean toward Enjoyer, Truster, Cooperator, and others in the left-hand column. In a relationship that squelches sexual desire, the roles are likely to lean toward those in the right-hand column: Wet Blanket, Doubter, Blamer, and so forth.

These roles can get ambiguous, though. For instance, if you identify as a Truster and Cooperator, are you really open, or are you saying "yes dear" only to please a partner, or keep the lid on a situation you fear might explode into rage or some other form of craziness. If you're an Empathizer, is that because you're more attuned to your partner than to yourself? Constant caretaking can drive a partner bananas, or enable destructive behaviors or addictions—with food, alcohol, or the Internet, for instance, or with other sexual partners. Conversely, you may see yourself as a Wet Blanket—when in fact your intent is to set appropriate boundaries or stand up for yourself.

From the columns on the next page, rank the roles that you think you play in your relationship. Then notice how you think these roles affect your desire for sexual connection. Again, there are no right or wrong answers.

Ask your partner to do this too. Then rank the roles you think each other plays. Then talk together—and listen carefully to one another.

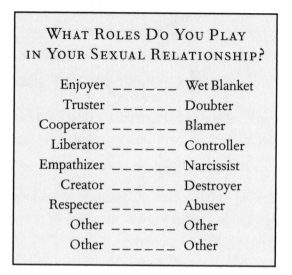

WHAT ROLES DO YOU PLAY
IN YOUR SEXUAL RELATIONSHIP?

Enjoyer	_____	Wet Blanket
Truster	_____	Doubter
Cooperator	_____	Blamer
Liberator	_____	Controller
Empathizer	_____	Narcissist
Creator	_____	Destroyer
Respecter	_____	Abuser
Other	_____	Other
Other	_____	Other

The basic question about assessing your sexual roles is: how can you enjoy all the good feelings that come from a sense of oneness without losing yourself in your partner? The dance of give-and-take may be different with different partners, and it may shift and change over time. No one formula fits all. But engaging mindfully in the dance is essential so that you can become more aware of the roles you're playing and more adept at communicating with yourself and your partner.

Reclaiming Your Sexual Desire
Using the ISIS Model to Help Fill Yourself Up

Recovering sexual desire involves all of you—body, mind, heart, and spirit—and all of your relationship, too. But in our just-say-no culture we're not encouraged to seek information about whole-person, whole-relationship sex. So most of us have to create our own routes to finding out who we are and what we want—and to remembering how to have fun, too. These may vary depending on our concerns, and our resources. There are many ways to create your routes. This section will show you how you can use the ISIS model to get started.

When sexual desire has taken a turn toward confusion, pain, and entanglement, I often ask clients to begin in the mental path of the ISIS Wheel.

This is the place where you can obtain a cognitive grasp of the situation and fill yourself up with knowledge.

EXPLORING THE MENTAL PATH TO DESIRE
FILLING UP WITH KNOWLEDGE

Sexual knowledge can be an antidote to fear, and an inspiration for desire. It involves much more than just being familiar with genital physiology and how to fit Tab A into Slot B—though of course that can help. When oneness with your partner seems to be the most erotically desirable thing in your world, it's crucial for you to understand without a doubt that the ways to get there are actually within you, not outside of you.

When you allow yourself to know that you're not powerless, you're not bad, and you're not the only one who feels the way you do, you may be able to relax enough to allow a whole new scene to unfold. You can begin the job of reclaiming sexual desire on your own terms so you don't have to acquire your good feelings secondhand, from someone else. Too many women spend their lives shopping in the wrong relational store—one that doesn't carry the kind of feelings that fit them.

Some women find it's helpful to work with a therapist or join a support group, especially if a relationship really does seem to be from hell. If substance abuse is involved, I always suggest that clients participate in twelve-step programs to supplement their one-to-one therapy. My personal journey included both Al-Anon groups (for partners of alcoholics) and ACOA groups (for adults who grow up in alcoholic families). Ultimately, several of us formed our own group, where we spent the better part of two years gently helping each other fill the gaps in our emotional education—like how to say what we wanted without behaving like a four-year-old having a tantrum. There was some painful trial and error, but also lots of life-changing information—and many laughs.

For other women, sexual knowledge begins with talking with your partner, and with your friends, too. You—and your partner—might also benefit from workshops that focus on relationship and desire. There are plenty to choose from, and they're all over the country. You can also take ISIS Connection workshops, or form your own group to discuss how integrating sexuality and spirituality affects your relationship and your desire. Find out about ISIS workshops and groups on my website: www. GinaOgden.com.

In addition, I encourage you to read, read, read. There are excellent books on sexual relationships, ranging from the joys of sensual pleasure to sacred sex to recovery from abuse, violence, and codependency. Whether you start your search at the bookstore or on the Internet, let yourself be guided by what appeals to you. Surveying what's out there is a good way to fill your gaps in information. For instance, did you know that relaxation and pleasure can produce the same boost in desire that you might get from taking hormone replacement therapy? You may have to read parts of many books to piece together this countercultural information. But let this search be part of your mental journey to desire.

Check out videos and DVDs too. The range extends from romantic erotica to raunchy porn. At the end of the last chapter we touched on the educational value of sexually explicit films. See which ones work for you— even if you have to set aside some of your prejudices about what is supposed to be tasteful, or move through your rage about how the porn industry treats women. The truth is, images of kissing and humping can actually jump-start flagging desire—and so can moving your anger. "Edges are often much more powerful than safe middles when the libido requires a jolt," says New York sex therapist Joy Davidson, author of *Fearless Sex*.

Sexy images can work for other species, too: "Porn Sparks Panda Baby Boom" proclaimed an Associated Press headline of November 27, 2006. Chinese zoo specialists found they could rev up erotic activity in clueless panda bears by showing them explicit films of their wilder fellows going at it in the bamboo forests. If explicit films work for pandas, maybe they're just the ticket for you. Seeing lust in action, and imitating it, might begin to refill your own wellspring of sexual desire—and relational wisdom.

EXPLORING THE PHYSICAL PATH TO DESIRE
PLAY LIKE A KID

Your adult experiences of sexual desire naturally tap into sensations and feelings you had as a child, whether your growing-up years were warm and sunny or stormy and miserable. Most of us had both kinds of weather in our childhoods, and all the climate changes you went through then can affect your feelings about sexual desire today. One concept sexologists tend to agree on is that we are sentient, sensual, sexual beings from the moment of our births. That's part of the definition of being fully alive.

You don't have to spend a decade in therapy to make connections with your past and share feelings about the present. There are many activities that can bring back your memories of childhood pleasure—or lack of pleasure. The "kid" activities I suggest below are all physical, but they can loosen your tongue—and hopefully a bunch of other tightly held parts as well. None of them is overtly sexual in the sense of "Hey baby, let's get it on!" But try them and see if they free up your communication skills and help generate sexual desire—or at least an understanding of what you might be holding back.

Play with your food. Peel an orange or a ripe mango and let the juice run all over your hands—maybe lick it off as you eat. Be creative. Be provocative. Imagine you're Eve plucking forbidden fruit. This association can connect you to your lineage of all the women in history as you plunge into your here-and-now senses.

Feed each other. Choose your favorite fruit (or lobster, or tofu, or whatever rings your bells) and feed each other Tom Jones–style with your fingers. Enjoy every slippery bite. Hot tip: if you do this outdoors it will help you connect sensual desire with nature, too. And the cleanup isn't so daunting. Another hot tip: When you do any of these exercises with a partner, make sure they're consensual. Hint: It is never sexually seductive to force food on someone. It's abusive.

Skinny-dip. This not only feels good, but it offers the taboo-breaking element of being naked out in the open. If there's no swimmable body of water nearby (or if skinny-dipping there will get you in trouble with the law or cause discomfort for others), you can slip into your bathtub together and play like porpoises—or into your shower and play like porpoises standing up. One of my favorite client couples—a dentist and his hygienist wife—had a distinctly hygienic approach to sex, which meant they weren't having that much fun in bed (which is what prompted them to see me). Their big breakthrough came on a road trip to visit their grown children, when they plunged naked into a pool at midnight at a name-brand inn, seemingly shedding their inhibitions along with their clothing. (OK, they broke a rule. I see it as divine intervention that they weren't caught.)

Play water baby. Go to a spa, a pool, or the wide ocean. You can wear a bathing suit with this one—or not, it's your call. You're going to float your partner in water, then you'll trade off and allow your partner to float you.

Ask your partner to lie back in the water. Then hold one hand under your partner's head and the other under the sacrum—at the base of the spine. Gently rock your partner back and forth in the water. Your partner's job is to breathe—and feel the sensations.

Whether you do this for five minutes or an hour, it can feel like floating in amniotic fluid—relaxing, balancing, rejuvenating, close to your partner, close to nature, close to God, Goddess, and whatever you hold dear. You'll likely feel trusting and grateful, way slowed down, ready to go deep with each other. If you want some special inspiration here, read Kenneth Ray Stubbs's innovative books on his "Secret Garden" approach to sex and sensuality, particularly his *Erotic Passions,* which is a guide to sensual bathing among other delights.

Exploring the emotional path to desire
Learning to say yes and no

When women talk about the emotional ups and downs of sexual desire, I find these often involve their feelings about saying "yes" and saying "no." Both words carry powerful medicine—and understanding them presents an opportunity for growth and healing, especially if you're in a relationship where there's some confusion about who's feeling what on behalf of whom.

"No" is about the power of control. It's about gatekeeping and boundaries. It's about preventing sexual interactions you don't want—like saying no to intercourse when you have a vaginal infection, or when you just don't feel up to opening up. Some women find that celibate periods—without any partner sex—can be a potent way to discover who they are, to experience their own sexual rhythms and deepest desires without filtering them through someone else.

"Yes" is about the power of opening—of lifting up the gates of feeling, making contact, sharing, acknowledging your own erotic desires. And sometimes in a wonderfully paradoxical way, saying yes is also about letting go. Letting go of the ingrained message that says "good girls don't." Or of the notion that you're too ugly, or too fat or thin, or too smart or dumb, or too whatever to be desirable. Or that you just don't deserve to feel this deliciously sensual. Saying yes isn't about giving up and giving in. It's not about being a pushover. It's about dissolving the barriers that keep you from knowing what you really want.

How might this actually play out in your relationship? Patti Britton, sex therapist extraordinaire and author of *The Art of Sex Coaching,* writes of a technique she calls the "positive sandwich." She says that an effective way to say no to what you don't want (like two-minute intercourse) is to reframe it into saying yes to something you do want (like more canoodling and kissing and emotional contact). Then you sandwich the yes message in with what you know already works for both of you.

Here's how the positive sandwich works. You start with what you know will get your partner's attention—you say something positive and true, like, "I love being with you, Harry (or Louise)."

Then you slip in your negative message—but you do it in a positive way. So it goes, "And even though I love making love with you more than anyone else in the world, I wish we could spend more time talking and kissing first."

Then you complete the sandwich by adding another positive statement that you know will work: "So, come over here for a big kiss, honey . . . I love you so much!"

Here, you've reframed what might be a big No into a big Yes for what you really want. "It works," says Britton.

If you're not sure how this positive sandwich might play out for you, begin by making a list of the kinds of sexual interactions you don't want—then make a list that reframes these actions into interactions you do want. It goes like this—I'll use Britton's example, then you fill in the columns with your own examples.

REFRAMING NO TO YES

WHAT I DON'T WANT	WHAT I DO WANT
Two-minute intercourse	Kissing, canoodling, and love
Write your examples here	Write your positive reframes here

It's all based on the simple principle that you're much more likely to get what you want if you offer a positive suggestion rather than a negative one. Try it—and keep trying until you create a sandwich that tastes good enough to enjoy every day.

Exploring the Spiritual Path to Desire
Wisdom from the Queen Bee and Other Forms of Nature

To treat yourself like true royalty you don't have to splurge on a pricey new outfit or a total makeover. Consider the queen bee, a creature of enormous energy and vitality. She lives some sixty times longer than her worker counterparts, and can lay up to three thousand eggs a day throughout her life span. Any beekeeper will tell you that what makes a queen a queen is that she feeds only on royal jelly, which contains high concentrations of everything that's good for you, and which is sweet as, well, honey.

What can we learn from the queen bee that will help us bring back sexual desire when it's gone missing? The learning can be summed up as: You are what you eat. I'm not talking only about physical nutrition. I'm talking about spiritual food, the royal jelly of our energetic body—call it *chi,* call it *prana,* call it life force.

You can fill yourself up with these energies just as surely as if you were attending to your physical diet. These energies are available everywhere. You can find them in nature. You can find them in music. You can find them when you exercise your body and your mind. You can find them in spiritual meditation and positive thinking. And like all your memories and "reruns," they affect your sexuality even when they're not specifically about sex.

Here's one way you can treat yourself like royalty. This is an exercise I use with individual clients. I also use it in my workshops, and even in lectures with hundreds of people attending. You can play gentle relaxing music to help set the tone—but it's not necessary. Just being present is all the setting you need.

TREATING YOURSELF LIKE ROYALTY
A MEDITATION

Breathe deeply and let yourself sit in the throne of your pelvis. Isn't that a great image? It was bestowed on me by my California colleague Sabine

Grantke-Taft, who travels all over the globe teaching a delicious process of trust and healing she calls "Radiant Embodiment."

When you are securely settled in the throne that is your own body, feel your energy expand to match your royal status. Remember that you are a queen. Remember that you are you. And remember that you are sexual.

If you want to take this into a broader visualization, imagine yourself sitting in the throne of your body—and also sitting in the lap of the Goddess who is holding you. I see her as the Great Mother, queen of the powerful realm of spirit—you can use any image that works for you. Queen bee, even. The important thing is to focus on breathing your enthroned self onto a sacred lap of safety and comfort where you are surrounded with unconditional love. As if you are feeding yourself spiritual royal jelly. Feel your energy continue to expand.

To take this visualization still further, imagine you are reaching out your arms to gather into your lap any part of you that's feeling especially vulnerable. This may be your wounded child-self, or your adult who's hurt or sad. Or it may be the "nice Nelly" part of you who works so diligently to keep things from falling apart. Hold this part of you with all the expanded energy you receive from the Great Mother who's holding you. This is the royal jelly of nurturance and support.

You can further your queenly stature by naming yourself as the goddess and the mother. I love the chant "Sacred Pleasure," by songwriter and performer Shawna Carol. It's from her CD *Goddess Chants*—and I often play it in my workshops.

> I am the Goddess. I am the Mother.
> All acts of love and pleasure are my ritual.

Repeating these phrases over and over can activate both your sexual desire and your spiritual power. As you chant or say this mantra, continue to hold yourself and be held. Feel yourself filling up. This is the royal jelly of expanded beliefs.

These simple visualizations can fill you up with your royal self. They can also help you let go of what may be keeping you stuck in the role of worker bee, drone, and codependent partner.

If you find yourself in a relationship from hell (or even not), I invite you to begin to release any unwanted energies you may be carrying for someone else. I mean right now, before you finish reading this page. Begin by breathing into the throne of your pelvis. It's from here that you expand into self-sufficiency—that place from which you can love and appreciate a partner, rather than feeling you're going to die without him or her.

This can be a powerful step away from depending on a partner for your sexual energy. More important, it's a step toward connecting with a universal source of energy that nourishes you, whether you locate that energy source in Goddess or God or a bee or a tree or the ocean or a work of art or something quite other. Give it any name that works for you. You can feed yourself with it. You can feed your relationship with it.

Drink in the life force, lap up the royal jelly, bathe in the *chi* and *prana*— there's plenty to go around. This is the fountain of desire. In this place you are the queen. You are the goddess. You are the mother. You are sufficient. All acts of love and pleasure surely can be your ritual.

7

ARE MEN THE PROBLEM?
Mars and Venus in the Bedroom

"WE NEVER HAVE SEX," complains Alvie Singer to his therapist in the movie *Annie Hall.*

"We're constantly having sex," says his girlfriend, Annie.

"How often *do* you have sex?" asks the therapist.

"Three times a week!" they reply together.

Most women in America have male partners—between 80 and 90 percent, according to contemporary surveys. If this is your story, understanding how men experience sexual desire is crucial to understanding how you experience your own. Even if you don't have a male partner (or any partner), knowing how men respond can help create a full picture for you as you seek to resolve the sexual journeys of your past and create new stories of what you want in the present—body, mind, heart, and soul.

But our usual language of desire tends to be one of separation, not education. It's centered around an age-old Mars-Venus debate, which locates men and women on opposing relational planets—a cosmos in which we have vast discrepancies in our sexual desire. Here, men dominate, women flirt, and relationships are driven by a need to control the sexual scene. It's Him vs. Her—like the perennial bickering about how often to have sex. We all know the locker-room litany. He wants intercourse, she wants love and romance. He wants oral sex, she wants eye contact. He wants it all the time, she seems to want it only on his birthday. It's a language that limits much of the popular conversation about sexual desire to scoring and Viagra jokes.

This opposite-sex mind-set shows up in sex research, too. There's a "didja come?" mentality that informs almost every big sex survey and sexual self-help book. It fuels a national desire to perform. It fuels a national anxiety about the potency men lose as they grow older. Performance-propping drugs net billions of dollars a year—almost enough to support a small war.

Think about how many e-mails you get offering instant enlargement for your penis. I get them even though I'm the proud owner of a vagina and clitoris. The gremlins in cyberspace haven't figured out that we aren't all men.

The truth is, our sexual desires are firmly embedded in how we're socialized as well as in who we are. The notion that women and men are opposite can show up as problems throughout our relationships—from who shops, does the dishes, and puts the kids to bed to who handles the family finances. Our methods of expressing our differences invariably extend to the bedroom. How do we get what we want? Through cluelessness? Through violence? Through submission? There are dominator men who think they know what women want without asking, without listening. And there are women who let them go on thinking that. It's a way of sex so entrenched in our social structure that it says as much about the culture as it says about individual men. In chapter 4 I introduced this idea as "cultural missionary position"—man on top.

Let's begin by looking at some of the gender stereotypes of sexual desire we all live with. The national assumption is that what makes men happy is genital stimulation and a postcoital cigarette. This is the picture we get from the media (well, these days maybe without the cigarette). We get it from commercials for Viagra and Cialis. We get it from sex surveys, which decade after decade keep asking the same questions about intercourse— how often, how "successful," and with how many partners.

According to the stereotypes, men are the sexual beasts, clawing at the gates. Women are the sexual gatekeepers who lack the erotic interest and know-how of men. These images are rooted in our history and they nag at us to this day—encoded in the language we use to describe sexual desire. The columns on the next page show some of the stereotypes.

Stereotypes are oversimplifications, to be sure. But they don't come from nowhere. Some women are indeed gatekeepers and some men do act like beasts, flaunting the kinds of dominator characteristics outlined in chapter 4. A well-heeled business executive recently came for an appointment waving the Mars-Venus argument like an American flag. Sex meant intercourse to him, and he was approaching it more like a drill sergeant than a lover. He claimed he had a right to sex with his wife anytime, anywhere, no matter what she wanted—because she was his wife. She had a story too, of course. She said she'd given in to this for going on twelve years, but now what she wanted was *out*—unless there was a big change in his approach. She felt he treated her like one of his possessions, not like a human being with ideas and feelings.

MARS-VENUS STEREOTYPES OF SEXUAL DESIRE

MEN'S DESIRE IS SUPPOSEDLY . . .	WOMEN'S DESIRE IS SUPPOSEDLY . . .
Initiative	Receptive
Assertive	Submissive
Physical	Emotional
Competitive	Cooperative
Genitally oriented	Whole-body oriented
Quick to arouse	Slow to arouse
Looking for sex	Looking for love
Focused on performance	Focused on connection

Ownership tactics like his aren't limited to American CEOs. They are globally alive in practices like marital rape, sexual slavery, and female circumcision. They are classically visible in the chador and burka that render a woman invisible to any man except her husband. And women have always been legitimate spoils of war. In some wars, women have been the ultimate prize, and even the reason for starting war. Gatekeeping tactics like the CEO's wife's were, and are, practiced by women everywhere. Often, refusing sex is the only way women can exert any measure of power and control in an impossible situation.

But Are Men Really the Problem?

In terms of women's sexual desire, some men are a problem, especially those like the client above who believe that women are the second sex. But let's also acknowledge that there are men who have come a very long way from the dominator mode. Or maybe it's that I've come a long way—from my feminist separatist days of the early 1970s, when sexism was next to racism and it seemed women had to fight for every inch of our bodies and our personhood. It's no wonder that the women's health book *Our Bodies, Ourselves* became an instant best seller back then—because it affirmed our rights to define our own sexuality, our own desire.

For me, one of the great surprises of my ISIS survey was the flood of positive responses from men—684 of them, ages eighteen to seventy-seven. Many wrote letters that seriously challenge the "real man" myths about performance and scoring. These men are undeniably "real." But they take sexual desire and relationship far beyond locker-room exploits and what sex educator Michael Castleman tactfully calls "all-genital love styles." Most of these men talk about sex in terms of connection, feelings, and meanings—just like the women who responded to the survey.

I probably had no business being surprised. I know men who do dishes, change diapers, march for world peace, and truly partner their wives and lovers in and out of bed. I know corporate executives who aren't focused on their penises, and who are empathic, thoughtful, caring, and open to change. Besides, I'd received a comeuppance about my own gender prejudices in the mid-1990s when I was first on the road with *Women Who Love Sex*. All manner of men came forth to say how moved they were to learn about the complexity—and spirituality—of women's sexual responses. Single men, committed husbands, widowers, and roving Don Juans (or as one man put it, "Don Wannabes"). My all-time favorite comment was from an elderly man at a book signing who confided: "You know, after hearing you talk, I think *I'm* a woman who loves sex!"

Gay men have moved me to look beyond the stereotypes, too, and also men in bisexual relationships. Their stories often take place in a climate of social ostracism, and also within the devastating legacy of HIV/AIDS. They underscore the need for finding our personal center when the world is falling apart around us, and of finding support in compassionate community. This is a need that in no way fits the macho "real man" image. Rather, it resonates with all too many women in this culture who are dealing with the ravages of poverty, abuse, and other forms of brutality.

I've learned that buying into Mars-Venus opposites seriously short-changes both women and men. For it doesn't allow for the vast range of individual motivations for sexual desire or the wide diversity in sexual expression. If you have another look at the lists above, you can see that we probably all bring some traits from both lists into our bedrooms, and beyond. We'll look more closely at this complexity a bit further on.

What Men Want

Let's talk about men whose private ways of being offer a broader picture of sexual desire, one that's rarely seen in public. Some 80 percent of the men who answered the ISIS survey say that what makes sex really satisfying is feeling loved and accepted. These men speak of sexual energy as "a powerful force of nature," not a personal "drive" that has to be instantly gratified or they're gonna die. They speak of "looking for unity-oneness-knowingness" and of "letting go of ownership/jealousy." This is not the old party line. In fact, some of the men who answered my ISIS survey sound so much like the women who answered that I've occasionally read out their responses and asked audiences to guess who's who. The truth is, our sexual similarities in being human often outweigh our sexual differences in being male or female.

Who are these men? A computer analyst who says he experiences as much hunger for connection with spirit as for physical contact with his partner. A carpenter who says intercourse isn't about competition and conquest, but about "commitment and reverence interwoven with the relationship." A high school teacher who reflects a powerful belief that sexual response is a path to realms where there is no separation of sex and spirit. He writes simply: "Sexuality is experiencing God."

A suburban realtor writes: "Conquests don't give the fulfilling experience that most men are led to believe, just a sense of control." He's referring not only to personal greed and violence but to the age-old custom of male ownership of women, which most of us know still exists although we'd like to pretend it doesn't. An electronics technician concurs, and takes the idea a step further. He suggests that how we conduct our intimate relationships can affect cultural well-being along with personal well-being: "Violence, over-restraint, and selfishness can create destructive sexuality. Used properly, sex can heal."

The meaning I gather from hundreds of responses like these from men all over the country is that sexual desire is powerful enough to take the war out of men just as it's been powerful enough to incite them to go to war. It's in the fluidity of sexual experience that men can move beyond their injunctions to dominate and control. They can let down their guards, allow themselves to feel vulnerable and tender. They can engage in a morality of empathy and love that carries over into everyday life. They can revel in their partners' deepest desires. To borrow a phrase from the poet Robert Frost, a sexual journey that begins in physical desire and delight can end in wisdom.

Some of the most moving descriptions of sexual connectedness are from older men. These are men who spent their formative years in the sexual dark ages of post–Great Depression America. So it's interesting that their later-life sexual attitudes soar so far beyond the two-minute average time for coitus that Kinsey reported in his 1948 survey of male sexual behavior. Perhaps these men discovered a new way of being during the freewheeling decades of the 1960s and 1970s. Or maybe they'd simply lived long enough to strip away some of their early conditioning and respond to their basic human needs for emotional and spiritual connection. Various studies show that human beings tend to become more spiritually focused as we age. So for a certain percentage of men, the aging process might generate a desire for intimate connection rather than a desire to keep replicating the ever-ready erections of their youth.

Most of the men who answered the ISIS survey take their searches for connection far beyond the intercourse model of sex. A retired social worker is one of many who affirm the ancient notion of sacred marriage for contemporary relationships—a dynamic we'll look at in chapter 12. I love his description of how he received a gift of sexual grace from Venus herself, the goddess of love.

> On February 12, 1994, my soul imploded with an incredible vision of a goddess during orgasm with my wonderful wife. This was not something I thought of or made up or created. I had no idea that this could, might, or would happen to anyone, let alone a man. Suddenly, in the center of my inner vision is

this lovely goddess, rising up from the ocean, so beautiful she broke my heart. I was not only beside myself with joy and rapture, I was also frightened, because she was real. I went back into therapy to help deal with her.

Like so many women who have talked with me, this man questioned his own sanity when found himself entering into conversation with a being from the unseen world. His perception that the goddess was *real* scrambled his entire belief system about time, space, and who's supposed to do what with whom, and where and when. Yet his goddess vision fits exactly into findings from contemporary brain research, which show that our sexual responses engage a multiplicity of the brain's systems—physiological, cognitive, emotional, spiritual—and cosmic as well.

Clearly, he experienced a spiritual awakening along with an expanded sense of sexual desire. Further, he says this vision transformed his life—and that it contained healing energy he was able to pass on to his clients before he retired from his practice.

Following her advent there was much synchronicity in my life. I feel even more love for women, and it seems that women feel this from me. I sometimes feel or "see" this goddess when I have eye contact with a woman—even someone I barely know. I know she is in all women. A few of my female clients have had archetypal visions shortly after beginning work with me, and I believe this is stimulated in part by a "downloading" of sorts, of this goddess moving through me in ways that are beyond my consciousness and ego. For me she represents the ultimate union of my sexuality and spirituality. She is a goddess and dropped in when my body was at its peak of sexual arousal.

Vive la Différence
And Our Similarities, Too

Witnessing men's responses to questions about the feelings and meanings of sex bears enormous significance for our full understanding of sexual desire. It strikes at the core of those Mars-Venus stereotypes that portray women and men as intrinsically different in the way we think, feel, and perform, and different in the nature of our erotic desire—what we want and how we want to express it.

Let's revisit the lists of gender stereotypes shown earlier in this chapter. This time, let's view them as a continuum of human complexities, rather than as a catalogue of built-in differences. Reframing these lists into a scale offers another method to help you assess your sexual desire—separately, and also with your partner. Whether you're a man or a woman, every item on the scale may be true of you, at least to some degree. For instance, you may be both genitally oriented and whole-body oriented. You may be both physical and spiritual, assertive and submissive, and on and on. Your task is to acknowledge where you are and what moves you sexually.

For each pair of statements on the scale below, check the line segment that's closest to the word that reflects your experience—and feel free to add other statements that are true for you. Notice whether or not your desire scale changes if you apply it to different partners or special circumstances—such as that first grope in the backseat of your dad's Buick, or perhaps your honeymoon (each of which I know from personal experience can run hot or cold).

DESIRE ASSESSMENT SCALE
MY APPROACH TO SEX IS PRIMARILY...

Initiative	_ _ _ _ _ _	Receptive
Assertive	_ _ _ _ _ _	Submissive
Physical	_ _ _ _ _ _	Emotional
Competitive	_ _ _ _ _ _	Cooperative
Genitally oriented	_ _ _ _ _ _	Whole-body oriented
Quick to arouse	_ _ _ _ _ _	Slow to arouse
Looking for sex	_ _ _ _ _ _	Looking for love
Focused on performance	_ _ _ _ _ _	Focused on connection
Other	_ _ _ _ _ _	Other
Other	_ _ _ _ _ _	Other

If both you and your partner fill out this scale, you might unearth some interesting news about your similarities and differences in sexual desire—and maybe shed light on some of those "special circumstances."

Do your similarities make you yawn—or do they attract you to one another? Do your differences drive you apart—or do they leave you happily humming *vive la différence?* Perhaps some of them move you to expand each other and your relationship. Remember that wonderful phrase from Fritz Perls I quoted earlier, "Contact is the *appreciation* of differences."

Exploring Your Sexual Desire
Using the ISIS Model to Become a More Conscious Lover

I cannot tell you how many women have asked me over the years, "I'm ready to expand my sexual desire—but how do I begin to talk about this with my husband, my boyfriend, my lover?" It occurs to me that the most effective way I can answer this question is to show you how I begin the conversation with male clients who are ready and willing to become more conscious and caring sexual partners. So I'm going to address some of the words that follow directly to men—as modeling for the women who are asking for guidance, and also as inspiration for the husbands, boyfriends, and male lovers who are reading this book. I typically start by giving men the same courtesy I give women—I frame the conversation in a way that removes blame and judgment. Here we go:

As a man, how do you learn to expand your desire for connecting in a whole person way instead of just on-and-off intercourse? It takes courage to change. Our national conversation about sex is all about "doing it"—the performance model. Intercourse and orgasm are the goals. And God forbid your erection should fall short. You risk being laughed at, rejected, losing your status as a real man. If you can't perform intercourse, then this model says you're dysfunctional. Or worse, impotent. This can be painful and humiliating. Impotence means you can't satisfy your partner. Impotence means loss of power. So let's start with some powerful new ways you can explore the physical path.

EXPLORING THE PHYSICAL PATH (ESPECIALLY FOR MEN)
NEW WAYS TO FIND PLEASURE AND BECOME AN IRRESISTIBLE LOVER

Boisterous boinking is not the only route to sexual pleasure. Really. If you think this is just a woman talking, remember what the men in this chapter have to say about the deep erotic pleasures of relationship. Then, if you want to learn about being a really spectacular lover, read the rest of the book and find out what women have to say, especially about the men in their lives—their versatility, their ability to express physical sex on an emotional and spiritual level.

Hot tip #1: Pay attention to her. Chances are, you'll find out at least a couple of important truths. One is that flashy lovemaking techniques may attract and excite, like a gorgeous display of male plumage. But what really satisfies is your intent, and your ability to join your energies with hers. When you're touching your partner, do you really *get* what she's feeling? That can count for more than a virtuoso performance.

What most women experience as great physical sex isn't about the size of your penis. It's more about the size of your heart and your imagination. It's about connection, trust, and your willingness to risk meeting her somewhere beyond your own physical and emotional comfort zone. It's about partnership—the sense of setting off on a sexual journey together into the unknown.

Hot tip #2: Develop a magic touch. See how far you can extend your range of physical touch beyond the usual "homing sites," such as her breasts and clitoris. How does she react when you place your warm hand on her abdomen and blow softly on her upper chest? Here, you're connecting her sexual center with her heart center. She may come to orgasm right in your hand! She'll think you're a sexual magician. And you will be. What about when you hold her against your chest with both of your hands between her shoulder blades and breathe in unison with her? This way, you're making heart-to-heart connection. See the chakra chapter in *The Heart and Soul of Sex* and experiment with how you can contact each of your energy centers with hers.

Wherever you focus, don't just grab and pluck at her body parts—remember the husband in an earlier chapter who rubbed his wife's clitoris as if he was Simonizing his car. Go slow. Go gentle. Or go fast and deep. But notice her. Feel her body respond to your touch. Feel her energy and notice how it affects yours. Ask her what she likes. Pay attention to all that she communicates to you, verbally and nonverbally. Masters and Johnson, who were the Adam and Eve of sex therapy, used the term "sensate focus" to describe this kind of body exploration.

And—very important—remember that the body doesn't stop at the surface of the skin. Every time you touch each other, your bodies respond to the intention and the meaning behind your touch, whether or not you're consciously aware of it.

Hot tip #3: Redefine "down there." One of the assignments I've given sex-weary couples is to make mad passionate love to each other for at least half an hour—but never to go above the ankles. That is, give each other the most sensual and intricate foot massages you can muster. Go wild—use your breath and tongue and hair as well as your fingers. The feet are filled with nerve endings that connect to every part of your body—you can find a reflexology chart on the Internet if you want to know exactly what these connections are (try www.reflexology-research.com, for example). But you don't need to become a pressure-point expert. All you need to know is that as you find more and more inventive ways to touch your partner, you're on your way to becoming an irresistible lover.

For more suggestions, have a look at the Extragenital Matrix at the end of this book, and also see the chapters on ceremony and Tantra in *The Heart and Soul of Sex*. These can begin to open you to new avenues of lovemaking. For more ideas still, see Michael Castleman's *Great Sex* and Ian Kerner's *She Comes First*. Both these books have received rave reviews from men—and women. Also read Thomas Moore's 1998 best seller, *The Soul of Sex*, which argues that sex is never only physical—it always involves the soul. All of these authors are *real men*. Their authenticity is impeccable.

Exploring the Mental Path (especially for women)
Expect More from the Men You Love

Now I want to address women—to dispel some of the gender mythology that surrounds sexual desire. If we get too locked into male-female differences, we can find ourselves trapped in defensive mode. Countless men have confided to me that they want more than the kicks that come from macho performance—the need for closeness and intimacy is part of being human, and part of being sexual, too. But countless men have also confided how difficult it is for them to break through their control issues to show these desires, or even feel them. Some men feel they're able to break through only during the act of intercourse—when pleasure overwhelms their iron-man conditioning. It's no wonder they're so hot to "do it" morning, noon, and night no matter what else is happening in their lives—or yours.

If the man in your life has been heavily conditioned never to show any form of vulnerability, he'll probably have learned how to separate his body from his heart and spirit. He may be in emotional and spiritual lockdown. If you expect instant intimacy, you'll be in for disappointment. You may have to guide him on exactly how to accompany you into your special mysteries of sexual desire. If he doesn't follow you all the way, back up and lead him slowly. Stop to smell the roses along the path. He may kick and scream at first, but in the long run you're doing both of you a favor.

Sure, it's his responsibility to figure out all these relationship complexities for himself. But if you care about him, give him a break. Power corrupts—and men have been in power for centuries. As I mentioned earlier, they're bucking a time-honored custom that says they can have sex with anybody, any old how, just because they *can*. In the Middle Ages, it was *droit du seigneur*, the right of the lord of the manor to have his way with any bride in the manor on her wedding night. Vestiges of this kind of male ownership are still around, although it's not necessarily tolerated in the way it used to be, even among our society's most powerful men. A notorious example in the 1990s was the "Zippergate" scandal that resulted when President Bill Clinton had his way with "that woman," a young intern. In his 2005 autobiography, Clinton finally, poignantly, admitted that this sexual boundary-dropping was in response to the privilege of male power—he'd done it just because he *could*.

Exploring the Emotional Path (also for women)
Wake Him Up by Asking for What You Want

Back to one of the ongoing mantras of this book: ask for what you want—even if it involves more emotion, more contact, more spirituality, more relationship. Asking is difficult for most women. Especially for those of us who've been socialized to take care of everybody else before we begin to think about ourselves. But where are we if we don't ask? We're stuck in perpetual cultural missionary position—possibly underneath a well-socialized man who's perfectly willing to stay on top.

So make your personal wish list—and keep updating it, because it's likely to change over time (more about this in the final chapter). Think about the kinds of sexual connection you really want from your husband, your partner, your lover. Maybe you want him to look profoundly into your eyes. Or listen to your deepest needs for love and approval. Or touch you with smart hands—in ways that turn you on, not ways he guesses turn you on. Or watch you pleasure yourself so he can learn how you like to be touched. Or shave off his beard so he doesn't prickle you during oral sex. Maybe you just want to drink in his male energy without having his male ego get in the way. Sip it into your chakras. Mmmm. Delicious.

Learn your pleasure ABCs. Your job is to know the emotional ABCs of sexual pleasure. (A) it's OK to want pleasure, (B) you deserve pleasure, and (C) it's OK to enjoy pleasure when it comes your way. So tune up your second and third chakras and go for it. As Dorothy learned in *The Wizard of Oz:* You *are* home. All you have to do is wake up!

Now that you know what's possible, don't allow the men you love to fall back into old patterns that leave you out. There's nothing wrong with a hot sweaty quickie. But don't let your husband separate physical sex from caring and meaning. Don't let your boyfriend assume you're satisfied just because *he's* kicking back with the proverbial cigarette.

You may have to help expand your man's horizons. Keep reminding him until he gets it on his own. Use language he understands. Humor may help—heart-opening humor, not sarcastic needling. Let him know that he can arouse your desire by listening to your feelings and appreciating your intelligence. Or that his cheerfully doing the dishes and laundry may be more of a turn-on than his Valentine's gift of peekaboo lingerie. The important thing here is to be real. And adapt your strategy to fit his reality, too—including his ethnic background and culture. A soul brother or a Latino is going to have different imagery than a dyed-in-the-wool WASP.

And if he doesn't get it, get serious. Let him know your needs are important and present. If he still doesn't get it, think about counseling—to create a safe place for you to discover whether your relationship is beyond redemption or if you just need some assistance with emotional communication. If he—or you—become enraged or abusive when you suggest changes in his sexual approach, it's definitely time to seek help—fast. The Resources section in the back of the book suggests how you can find a counselor in your area, and also how to locate an abuse hotline.

Exploring the spiritual path (for both women and men)
Men and women changing the mold

As a woman and as a therapist I want to end this chapter by speaking to both men and women from my heart. Following the ISIS paths can change your life—to become more sexually satisfying, more meaningful, more intimate. It can do even more. It can help counter the clichés that girls and women learn at their parents' knees about how men only want One Thing—and we all know what *that* is, heh, heh, heh. It can help counter the locker-room messages boys and men learn about possessing and scoring.

I say this from personal experience as well as from having worked with many couples in the course of my career. Men can be infuriatingly creative in finding ways to keep themselves from intimate contact. In my family of origin, they did it by making jokes. It was a skill they developed to an art form. But it had its intimacy drawbacks. It wasn't until my father was dying and in a coma that I was able to say "I love you" without some kind of witty comeback from him that deflected my deep wish to connect with him. And until my late thirties I kept choosing male partners who were similarly stuck in their heads, responding to old tapes and messages and jokes about how real men shouldn't show feelings.

Don't let this degree of distancing happen to the man in your life—and don't let it happen to you. Lovers don't let lovers slip off the ISIS paths. Keep expecting more openheartedness, more intimacy. If he pleads cluelessness, don't allow him to hide under a rock of not-getting-it. Keep feeding him the clues until he gets your message. Ask him to remember how he felt when you and he first met—and keep pushing for details. Revisit his deeply felt dreams with him—and see where they match your dreams—or

94

excite new dreams for you. Be innovative. A counselor colleague asks clients to watch the 1989 film *Shirley Valentine,* in which a disaffected British housewife finally lures her workaholic husband to a Greek Island to enjoy a sunset with her. Maybe the transformation this couple experiences will speak to you.

You can't change a partner who doesn't want to change. But you can change yourself—and enjoy the results. I love how holistic physician Christiane Northrup phrases this truth in her wildly popular 2007 PBS special on the wisdom of menopause. She begins by saying: "The best predictor of great sex is a new partner." Then she completes her statement by creating an all-important clause about self-care and self-responsibility: "So it's up to you to *become* that new partner."

Becoming a new partner means you understand that the most effective sexual foreplay in the long run is fairplay with your partner. Men, this means you recognize her as the glorious, magical human being that she is—every day, not just after the Sunday ballgame is over and you want to make out. Women, this means you recognize him as the hero he is—every day, not just after he fixes the busted screen door and chases the spiders out of the basement. Sexual fairplay is love in action. To my mind, it has implications far beyond our individual sexual relationships. It offers hope that equal power balances between women and men may someday be a reality.

A commercial artist offers this prose poem he addresses to his artist wife. It embodies the co-creative principle underlying the partnership notion of sexual relationship—and the ancient notion of the sacred marriage of gods and goddesses. It illustrates that co-creativity can exist in our human lives—as an integral part of our sexual desire.

To a Goddess:
You provide me a forum for expression.

When I'm with you art comes alive! Images take form. Creativity is at its best.
"Magic" is not just a word to describe something we are mesmerized by . . . it becomes an entity, in and of itself. We can touch and taste it.

"Spirituality" is not just a word to describe a feeling . . . it has become an important part of my "real" world.

Through my feelings of spirituality I am able to heighten my senses and touch places otherwise unknown.

You are my audience—and my partner!

And of course my teacher and my pupil!

"Ceremony" has been very kind to us. It can simply be a "look." It can be one candle. It can be the sharing of breath. It can be aroma, or what we wear, or where we are, or how we touch. Any one or all at once—it doesn't matter. We are able to follow the direction of our desire. We both truly care how the other receives, responds, is pleased, and is comfortable in every way.

As powerful as I sometimes feel—I am humbled by the strength of your sweetness!

And because of all these things

I realize that we have just begun . . .

From a God.

8

BRINGING UP BABY

Desire Changes and Challenges after Childbirth

Y OU HAVE A NEW BABY. You are tired. You've made it through labor and delivery, which was challenging enough, and now you're up day and night with your newborn. You have morphed from an independent adult who calls the shots into someone you hardly recognize. Who is this woman lurching around in slippers, leaking from just about every orifice, and what is this new chapter in her life? Sexual desire feels like something that used to happen to somebody else—a woman you vaguely remember as vibrant and playful and ready to make love until dawn.

What's wrong with this picture? Why do new moms—and some seasoned moms, too—so often turn away from the very sensual and sexual urges that created their babies? Bringing children into this world is a miracle, the ultimate generative act. But it introduces changes and sometimes challenges to every aspect of our lives, including our capacity for sexual response and intimacy.

Let's begin with the basic understanding from earlier chapters that sexual desire is complex. It involves much more than just your physical sensations. Sexual desire also involves your emotions—how you feel about your partner, about being a mother, and about the postpartum moods that burst upon you like flash floods. Sexual desire involves your thinking—your beliefs and messages about sexual partnership and about how kids should be raised. Sexual desire involves your spiritual capacity—your yearning for deep connection and meaning with yourself, with your partner. At its most intense, sexual desire contains joys and wonders beyond words—and it can also plunge you into an abyss of loneliness and despair. The process of pregnancy, birth, and mothering tends to amplify any and all of these states.

Many women have shared with me how difficult it's been for them to revive desire for sex after childbirth. I can relate. The birth of my first baby marked a descent into an abyss. My son was delivered by a surprise Cae-sarian section—surprise because my doctor was arrogant enough not to inform me that a surgical delivery was probable, and because I was compli-ant enough not to ask questions. This was 1961, before *Our Bodies, Our-selves* and other blessings of the women's health movement. Doctors gave little information or counseling during pregnancy or afterward. Although it was the cusp of the sexual revolution (the birth control pill was intro-duced in 1962), mothers were routinely left out of the childbirth loop. We were patronized, sedated, and left with no shred of sensuality intact.

I arrived home with a wonderful nine-and-a-half-pound son, an inch-wide scar up the middle of my belly, and abdominal spasms that produced monumental gas. Intimate contact was painful and embarrassing. Much more important, I was in emotional shock. I felt I'd failed utterly. Failed to have a "natural" birth. Failed in my role as wife and mother. Postpartum depression, or "baby blues" as it was called then, couldn't begin to describe my ongoing terror that I'd somehow leave the baby behind in the grocery store or let him tumble out our tenth-story apartment window. Sex? It was out of the question. Not only was there all that gas, but what I really craved was sleep and for my son to live through his infancy despite my ineptness. My husband and I lacked the communication skills to talk about the kinds of closeness and support we needed back then, and that marriage did not survive.

Not every mother suffers this depth of disconnection of course, though I usually see some nods of recognition whenever I tell this story. Some women bloom when they become mothers, and their sexual desire blooms, too. But whatever your experience of birth and bringing a baby into your life, your relationship with your partner is bound to become drastically complicated. Baby care is demanding. Your longing for sleep may win out over your longing for sex. Holding and cuddling your baby may fill your need for closeness and touch. So if sexual desire drops off your radar screen, you're not alone—it occurs for many new moms though the exact percentage is unknown.

When will desire return? Every woman's timetable is unique, and it can vary from one birthing experience to another. Conventional wisdom says it takes at least six full weeks to physically recover from giving birth. For some women it may take much longer, though. It depends on your age. It depends on your physical, emotional, and spiritual well-being. It depends on what your childbirth experience was like. It depends on your nutrition, your hormone balance, and how rested you are. It depends on the empathy between you and your partner. Some women are hot for intercourse long before the recommended six-week waiting period is up; others may need a year or more. Some women want to get pregnant again right away, others can't believe they ever put their bodies through all that and never want to risk going through it again.

The return of desire after childbirth also depends on whether you've come to terms with your own history. Was there nurturing in your child-hood—or was there disappointment and abuse? Having a child will bring up feelings about your own early life. This can be one of the blessings of motherhood, even if those feelings are difficult ones. Our children can wake us up, helping us see what emotional baggage we're carrying around. In fact, bringing up baby can bring up all the unresolved issues of your past and magnify them until you absolutely have to pay attention. In terms of desire and all other issues too, it's crucial that you listen to your body, mind, heart, and spirit and recognize where *you* are in the healing process. Six weeks is not a magic marker.

Your Postpartum Hormones and How They Affect Desire

The word "hormone" comes from the ancient Greek for "stir up" or "set in motion." Postpartum brings a new hormonal landscape to your sexual relationship—and this landscape may constantly shift and change. Let's look at some of what we know about the hormonal changes after preg-nancy and birth and how they affect your sexual desire. Note how your own experience matches the descriptions below, or departs from them.

OXYTOCIN

Oxytocin sets your loving feelings in motion. When you gaze adoringly into the tiny features of your baby, and melt when those little hands explore your skin, you've definitely fallen in love. This is one of nature's strokes of genius—at least for most mothers. The baby needs you, and your body releases hormones that draw you to your baby. Oxytocin delivers a further bonus for mothers who breastfeed. It triggers uterine contractions that can feel divine and make those dusk-to-dawn feedings worth every minute of lost sleep—more about these midnight pleasures a bit further on.

PROLACTIN

Prolactin is another hormone that's released during breastfeeding, and it triggers feelings of satisfaction and contentment. The release of prolactin might account for a drop in sexual interest during the breastfeeding period. This hormone is also released following orgasm—and it makes you feel as if you've just had sex. The particular function of prolactin is to flood you with a sense of well-being and "enough"—which means a natural relaxation of your desire for sexual stimulation. It's the hormone that tells you it's time to roll over and enjoy a deep relaxing sleep. And since you're constantly sleep deprived as a new mother, you're more than happy to answer its call.

ESTROGEN

Estrogen triggers vaginal lubrication. Its levels temporarily decrease after childbirth, and you may find that your vagina isn't quite as juicy as it used to be, until your estrogen decides to kick back in. Some women say intercourse feels as if they're being sandpapered—not a sensation that leaves them calling out for more. If dryness is a factor in your postpartum sex, try using a lubricant—most sex therapists recommend Astroglide, which is water-based and long-lasting. Or saliva, which doesn't require a trip to the store. Note that saliva's also naturally warm, and a talented partner can apply it to you by mouth.

THYROID

Thyroid helps regulate your moods—and a host of other things too. Your thyroid levels may decrease after childbirth—so if you feel exhausted, depressed, bitchy, and fuzzy-brained, if your formerly glossy hair's falling out, and you can't take off the fifty pounds you packed on during pregnancy, you're not necessarily going crazy. But your thyroid may be temporarily out of whack. It's time for a trip to the doctor. A simple blood test can determine low thyroid, and some temporary medication will most likely get you over the hump. If pills aren't your thing, you can seek other ways to get back into balance. For some women the shift back to feeling human comes with a combination of acupuncture, homeopathy, nutritional supplements, meditation, TLC, and, yes, uninterrupted sleep.

Body Image and Other Scary Subjects

A friend complained that even though her baby is a year old, she still feels like a beached whale. Looking in the mirror makes her cry. It doesn't take rocket science to understand that loss of self-image can mean loss of sexual desire, or fear that your partner won't find you alluring any more. Who wants to cuddle up to someone who's busting out of her jeans, smells of sour milk, and sobs during meals? Or whose passion is totally focused on a little person in Pampers? It's crucial that you and your partner communicate so that you're on the same page about what's happening. It can be scary to bring up the subject if you think you're the only woman who's ever felt that way, though. It may help to hear from some other women who've been there. Hint: call up a few friends who've been through it.

YOUR BREASTS

You may find that your breasts are exquisitely arousable after childbirth. Or you may keep them swaddled in a heavy cotton bra because they're way too swollen and tender for a lover's touch. If you're nursing, your nipples may crack and bleed at first. You may also feel your breasts don't belong to you any more—they belong to the baby. "They're just a couple of Good Humor wagons for my son," said one woman. "They dribble and squirt whenever he cries."

The other side of the coin is that you may find breastfeeding to be highly erotic. This doesn't mean you're some kind of pervert who gets her jollies from infants. It means you're experiencing one of nature's gifts to nursing mothers—and it's my fervent hope that you allow yourself to enjoy every minute of it rather than feeling wracked with confusion and guilt. Here's the sequence of what happens. When your baby sucks your nipples, this releases oxytocin—the "love hormone" you met earlier. This triggers uterine contractions designed to bring your uterus and vagina back into shape. These contractions can feel just as good as orgasms. Well, they *are* orgasms. And they *do* feel good. They're just not stimulated with sexual intent. You also get a rush of prolactin, mentioned earlier, which helps send a sigh of relaxation through your body and put a smile of contentment in your heart.

YOUR VAGINA

Will your poor overworked vagina ever recover from birthing a baby? Will it be too slack for satisfying intercourse? Some women worry about this. But rest assured. The tissue of your pelvic floor is highly elastic and will most likely spring back to pre-birth form, or very close—another of nature's gifts to new mothers. To speed this process and also help make your vaginal canal more responsive to pleasure for you and your partner, you can do Kegel exercises, which I'll describe later in this chapter.

But first, a word about vaginal surgery: You may hear from some "makeover" commercial that maybe a "little tuck" in your vaginal wall would be a good way to get your vagina back into shape. Be wary. Unless you had extensive tearing during delivery, you don't need plastic surgery. And if extensive tearing did occur, then it would require more than just a little tuck. And any vaginal surgery is bound to create scar tissue that will reduce sensation for you.

As I outlined in chapter 1, the unhappy truth is that there's an age-old obsession with altering the size and shape of women's genitals. In our North American culture, we don't condone infibulation (suturing shut the vaginal opening) or clitoridectomy (cutting out the clitoris). But we do set standards for facial beauty and breast size, and now there are standards being set for the beauty and size of our vulvas—our vaginal opening, lips, clitoris, the whole works. Vaginal surgeries are marketed to women who feel they aren't good enough or attractive enough—and to women who have time and money (and pain tolerance) for cosmetic projects beyond pedicures and waxing.

I'm not knocking the real miracles made possible by today's surgeons and plastic surgeons, but I do urge you to appreciate your own genitals in all their unique glory—and to think critically if anyone suggests you should change "you" into what they think "you" *ought* to be like.

YOUR ORGASMS

Some women say they're more easily orgasmic after childbirth. Perhaps this is because motherhood helps them feel lush and confident. Perhaps it's because the G spot on the front wall of the vagina has been awakened as the baby's head progressed through the vaginal canal. Whatever the reasons, if this is your story, accept this gift from the goddess of good fortune and enjoy each and every orgasm as fully as possible.

If you're not more orgasmic, or if you haven't ever experienced an orgasm, it's never too late to explore your potential. As I point out in *The Heart and Soul of Sex*, the paths to your orgasms may be complex—and deeply embedded in your relationship or your past history. Or they may be literally at hand, through the pleasures of masturbation. The acknowledged queen of hand and vibrator is sexologist Betty Dodson, and her *Sex for One* has helped two generations of women find the path to their first orgasm and many more. Now *that* book is an inventive gift for the new mom who already has more teensy outfits than her baby can possibly wear.

Traumatic Births

Childbirth isn't always easy. There are countless ways it can be traumatic, from Caesarean section, episiotomy, vaginal tears, massive hemorrhoids, and worse. If your baby is born with a disability, your entire life can stop—for months or forever. A whole set of other traumas may arise from the invasive procedures of in vitro fertilization or the tortuous procedures of adoption. Any and all of these take time to heal. Not only the physical scars, but the emotional and spiritual ones as well. Some women come through these kinds of experience enraged at their doctors, lawyers, and anyone else in their path. Or like me, they feel like failures and can remember only the pain and out-of-control scenes of childbirth, not the joy. All of this takes a toll on desire.

It is not the scope of this book to plumb the depths of traumatic birth experiences, but they need to be acknowledged. If there's been birth trauma for you or for your baby, you and your partner need to communicate with each other more than ever—talking, holding, helping, allowing grief to flow—and eventually allowing your sensual feelings to resurface and replace the numbness that so often comes when events lie too deep for tears. I invite you to seek all the counsel and support you can find.

"Passionate Birth"

At the other end of the spectrum from traumatic birth is passionate birth—a subject I learned a great deal about in 2007, when I had the pleasure of chairing a doctoral dissertation committee for the Institute for Advanced Study of Human Sexuality. The student was Danielle Harel, a seasoned childbirth educator and sex and intimacy coach. Her dissertation was an exploration of orgasmic childbirth, a subject that's not been systematically studied before in this way, and she's given me permission to include her work in this chapter.

Two major scenarios emerged from Harel's data. One was what she called "unexpected birthgasm." These are surprising orgasms women experienced at the moment of birth. They occurred without any sexual stimulation or fantasy, and the women she interviewed didn't interpret them as especially *sexual*—just as a very big surprise. A physiological explanation for this phenomenon may be that when the baby's head descends into the birth canal it puts pressure on the hypogastric and pelvic nerve systems, which can induce physical orgasms as a woman delivers.

The other scenario Harel found was what she termed "passionate birth." Here, women chose to incorporate their sexuality openly and intentionally during labor. This goes light-years beyond the usual medical practice of treating childbirth as a disease that requires hospitalization and pain medication. All of Harel's interviewees had uncomplicated deliveries and healthy babies. Aside from these crucial points, four major factors contributed to their passionate births.

1. These women enjoyed vital sexual relationships with their partners and had a thorough understanding of birth—its physiology, emotions, and meanings. They (and their partners)

considered childbirth to be a natural part of the sexual spectrum, and they incorporated massage, kissing, and masturbation into the birthing experience.

2. Instead of bracing against labor pains or dulling them with anesthesia, these women used sexual stimulation to ease their contractions. Some of the women experienced contractions as intensity rather than pain. One woman commented afterward, "They're called contractions but I felt them as expansion."

3. They established a safe, private environment in which to give birth. They created the setting, included midwives who believed in the idea of passionate birth, and decided who else was going to be present—sometimes no one, and sometimes friends and family members.

4. Their partners played a crucial role in supporting and creating passionate birth experiences for these women. They held, supported, and pleasured them, and welcomed their babies into the world.

Clearly, not every couple is able or willing to enter into a full-blown passionate birth experience. But Harel's work says to me that some degree of passionate birth is worth contemplating for almost any prospective parents. Even in a hospital setting childbirth can be more human and sensual if you can adopt some of the attitudes mentioned above—instead of seeing your birth experience as a medical procedure filled with apprehension and pain.

But let's not set up passionate birthing as yet another standard for women to achieve. Women already have enough to live up to. Perhaps it's enough for us to know that there can be positive outcomes if you experience childbirth as part of the sexual spectrum. These particular women reported feeling more "womanly" and "ripe" postpartum, and infinitely appreciative of their bodies' ability to deliver a baby in pleasure, not pain. Some referred to their births as the most intimate experience they'd ever shared with their partners. Perhaps most important, they carried their intimate feelings postpartum to their partners—and their babies.

Exploring Your Sexual Desire after Childbirth

Using the ISIS Wheel to Deepen Intimacy

Here are some ways you can practice whole-person intimacy after child-birth, while also nurturing yourself.

DEEPENING YOUR PHYSICAL INTIMACY
BREATHE, BATHE, CUDDLE, "KEGEL"

My first suggestion is a simple one: *Breathe together.* You're going to breathe anyway, so why not enjoy the process, and use it to connect with your partner? A delightful way of doing this is to spoon breathe—maybe to some totally relaxing music. Snuggle up behind your partner so you're like a couple of spoons in a drawer, with your breasts and belly pressed against his back and your arms around him so your hands are over his heart. (You can adjust this to fit your differences in size and shape, and you can roll over and reverse positions at any time.) Then match the rhythm of each other's breathing. You can do this for a few minutes or for an hour or more. You may fall asleep this way and wake up in each other's arms. If you decide to do three-person spoon breathing with your baby, note that babies inhale and exhale more rapidly because their lungs are still tiny—so don't try to speed up your breathing to match. Also, for safety's sake, take care not to hold your baby between the two of you.

Bathe or shower together. This means more than getting clean, though cleansing is an important part of physical intimacy. It's also a way to con-nect through water, which is a powerful conductor of energy. For some couples it's a way to play like children—a fabulous outlet for people who've taken on the awesome responsibilities of parenthood.

Cuddle. Let yourselves be sensual without a goal of intercourse. Hug, kiss, hold hands, give back rubs and foot rubs, cuddle on the sofa, sniff each other's hair, nibble each other's earlobes, ogle each other the way you did on your first date. These are all ways of reestablishing sensuous contact and letting each other know that your bodies still respond to one another.

Kegel. Take time to reclaim your body for yourself, too. Have a mas-sage, get a haircut, take an uninterrupted shower, do Kegel exercises—

named for Los Angeles gynecologist Arnold Kegel, who developed them in the mid-twentieth century. Basically what you do is tighten and relax your pubococcygeus muscle, or "PC" muscle (it's located in your pelvic floor) as if you're stopping the flow of urine, then letting it go. But don't think about urine. Think pleasure. Think elasticity. Think beautiful body. Think taking charge of your own health and well-being. The more Kegels you do the sexier you may feel. And you can do them anytime, anywhere. Try some now—even a few can help, and experts say you can do up to 150 per day. There's also a great deal of Kegel information on the Web—try www.childbirth.org.

Deepening Your Emotional Intimacy
Make Dates, Accept Help, Housebreak Your Partner

Make regular time together. Set intimacy dates with your partner—once or twice a week if you can. The time you spend together doesn't even have to be sexual, say some mothers, but these dates can set the stage for sexual expression when you're ready. I know moms who fiercely protect these dates as times to let go of the tensions of the day and share feelings—joys and hopes, resentments and fears. One mother says, "We listen to each other, even when we think we're too tired to hear one more word."

When talking doesn't do it for you and sex play seems more effort than you can muster, try this simple exercise: Sit opposite each other, place your right hands on each other's hearts, and breathe together—until you're breathing in unison. You may find this connects you energetically without having to speak. This is the basis of a Tantric technique designed to bring together body and spirit, man and woman, lover and lover.

Creative time management can help, too. As one harried mom reported to me: "You have to shift your perspective. There's just too much to do. I plan to vacuum my house when my twins go off to kindergarten—or maybe college." This woman has opted for sanity and relationship rather than perfect housekeeping, which can save a lot of heartache in the long run.

Accept help. If you can't live with household chaos, by all means, accept help. If you feel guilty about letting others do some of your cooking, cleaning, and childcare, remember that women have helped other women from the beginning. In other times and cultures we had the village. Babies and children belonged to everyone. New mothers got to be pampered in a special hut. A century ago we had the extended family, with at least three live-in generations to share the work. Now we have conveniences like microwaves and takeout food—as well as a far greater chance that you and your baby will survive the birth process. But too many of us lack a sense of caring community. So let others pitch in. If they didn't want to help you, they wouldn't offer. Some people just plain like to be around babies.

Housebreak your baby's father. Suppose your baby's father won't share? Even though some men are natural caretakers, others shy away from intimate relationships with their children, especially their babies. A story I hear too often is: "Yes, I have a husband, but when it comes to childcare I might as well be a single parent." I believe this is because too many men are conditioned to feel threatened by events they can't control. Your baby's father may have been frightened by witnessing the baby emerging from your vagina. He may be scared he'll break the baby if he picks it up. And he may simply have been brainwashed to think of childcare as "women's work."

All this can give rise to anger, even outrage, at the double standard that perpetuates men having the fun and women doing the work. How come *your* life changed so completely after the baby came but your husband is free to come and go just as he always did? Why hasn't *his* life turned upside down too? Is it that he just doesn't care enough to pay attention to the baby?

The truth is, the double standard is entrenched. Your baby's dad may care deeply but be at a loss as to how to show it. The immediate task is for you to set aside as much of your outrage and resentment as you can, and find ways to invite him to participate. You may have to be creative. You may also have to let go of your need to control every aspect of childcare and allow him to learn on the job. He may do a few dumb things with baby food or diaper changes. But imagine what might happen once he begins to take initiative. He'll start to be a real father. And (an added benefit) you'll have some time for yourself. Aha! Time for yourself means you can summon up your outrage again and focus it on changing the double standard in the culture—if this is what moves you.

On the desire front, seeing your partner connect lovingly with your baby can be a huge turn-on. Besides, many mothers need this kind of empathy and support with childcare before they can even begin to think about being sexual.

Speaking of empathy, there is an extraordinary phenomenon called "empathic pregnancy" that can create some hormonal magic in fathers, too, way beyond mere sharing and caring. Some new fathers actually experience a release of oxytocin that causes them to lactate (oxytocin is the "love hormone" you met earlier). They may not be able to take over breastfeeding responsibilities, but they can experience what it's like to suckle their babies. Lactation empathy can also occur for lesbian couples, and some have reported that both partners are happily able to share the breastfeeding.

Deepening your mental intimacy
Examine your beliefs, find sex-positive stories

This is a time to examine your beliefs about motherhood and life after motherhood—and to share them with your partner. Here are three questions you can ask yourself—and talk about with your partner. Doubtless you can think of many more.

1. Do you think you're the only one who's supposed to care for the baby—or is it OK to share this role with your partner? Sharing childcare may mean learning to relax your standards about the one right way to do everything from midnight feedings to washing dishes. But don't make assumptions, talk this over with your partner.

2. Do you believe childbirth has ruined your looks and your sex appeal? A mom who came to one of my workshops says she's developed a magic mirror—so she can look beyond her surface and straight into her big warm heart. Many women tell me that their minds and hearts expand with motherhood—wide enough to find more compassion for themselves. When you can connect with your compassion, you'll be more desirable to yourself—and probably to your partner as well. Check it out.

3. Does motherhood mean you're not supposed to be sexual anymore—or is it possible for you to be both a loving mom and a
vibrant sexual partner? Some cultures put mothers on a ped-
estal and endow us with an aura of divinity. In Latin cultures
it's called *marianismo,* after the Virgin Mary—full of grace,
the ultimate mother, in whose name women are supposed to
bear child after child to overcome the guilt of sexual pleasure.
In Anglo North American culture, too, it's not entirely OK
for mothers to have sexual feelings. Only a couple of months
ago I was asked to speak to a local mother's group about sexual
intimacy after children. The mothers turned out in force and
couldn't wait to start sharing. But the organizers had a tough
time publicizing the event. Both the local Fox News affiliate
and the *Boston Globe* refused to mention it. They said the subject was "too racy."

News flash! Motherhood is not sainthood—and this is
your chance to break with that myth if it holds any charge for
you. If you need another set of myths to fall back on, you can
always cite the really early traditions of lusty goddesses, like
Isis, whose divinity—and motherhood—were both rooted in
sexual pleasure.

DEEPENING YOUR SPIRITUAL INTIMACY
SHARE WISHES, DREAMS, AND EDUCATION FOR YOUR CHILDREN

Spiritual intimacy means more than sharing the same religion, though for
some partners this is vitally important. Even if you don't attend formal
services, you can develop a spiritual practice together or resume one that
you may have let slide. Your personal practice can be as simple as consciously thanking each other for being present in each other's lives. Or you
may create a sacred space in your home—perhaps to keep photographs
or flowers or other special items. How can this reignite sexual desire? It
brings intention and action together. It helps you remember who you are
in relation to yourself, your partner, and the universe.

Share with your partner. Mostly, the spiritual intimacy that ignites desire
means connecting with your partner in meaningful ways. It means talking

together about how it feels to be a family rather than a couple. It means sharing your wishes and dreams. It means sharing your frustrations, too. Maybe you both feel overwhelmed with work and exhaustion. Maybe you're concerned that one of you is distant from your kids, or attached in an overly sticky way. The point is, you can allow parenting to drive you apart—or you can use it to deepen the bond between you, creating opportunities to update what you really want.

Connect sexuality and spirituality. Spiritual intimacy may include deep discussions about the kinds of sexuality education you want for your family. Many of us have been taught that sex and spirit are separate. And we've been told it's immoral—and unhealthy—to display any shred of sexual feeling in the presence of our children. But think about this for a moment. Where else are your kids going to learn about love and intimacy? The truth is, they're going to see sex everywhere—more than three-quarters of network TV shows reportedly have some sexual content, and all bets are off once your kids learn to use a computer. Do you want them to take all their cues from television and cyberspace, where they may witness sex in the context of control or violence? As parents, you have the prime opportunity to model loving sexual values for your kids as they're growing up. Think of this kind of modeling as an investment in their relational intelligence and ability for connection.

By modeling sexual values, I absolutely do *not* mean using your children as sexual objects—that's abuse. Nor do I mean you have license to make out with your partner at the family dinner table to show your kids how Mommy and Daddy (or Mommy and Mommy) do it. But I do mean that it's also damaging to pretend sex doesn't exist. I can't tell you how often I've heard clients trace their sexual problems back to parents who seemed to have no erotic energy for one another. Or to walking in on "sexless" parents twisted in the throes of hot sweaty orgasm—which can seem like a life-and-death struggle when a child has no preparation.

I'm talking about age-appropriate stages to model what feels good, comforting, affectionate, and fun. Some new parents start right away with the family bed—sometimes sleeping alongside their kids for years. Granted, this is not everybody's cup of tea. But sharing sleeping space with children is typical of how families live in much of the rest of the world. For a smart discussion of sexual development from infancy to middle school, see *From Diapers to Dating: A Parent's Guide to Raising Sexually Healthy Children* by Debra Haffner—a mother, minister, and former executive director of the Sexuality Information and Education Council of the United States. Robie Harris has written some wonderful sex education books for children that are great for parents, too—and they're illustrated. My favorite is *It's Perfectly Normal: Changing Bodies, Growing Up, Sex, and Sexual Health.*

Invoking Baubo the "Belly Goddess"

When all's said and done, bringing up baby is a complex and imperfect art. Sometimes the way to keep your own sexual energy alive is through a sense of humor. I love the story of Baubo, the bawdy goddess whose special talent was to make women laugh during childbirth and other stressful situations. Versions of this goddess have appeared in various cultures from earliest history—joking, dancing, whirling, lifting her skirt, flashing her vulva, and generally reminding women of our generative power for life, love, movement, and sexual desire. This belly-baring ancient one is an archetypal embodiment of sex and spirit. You'll find her in Paleolithic caves and Indian temples. You'll find her in French cathedrals—as one of the pagan fertility symbols that abound even in these Christian strongholds. You'll find her in Irish chapels—as the carved Sheela-na-gig squatting naked over the door. She defies cultural no-nos by defining the entrance to sacred space. Her vulva is the doorway, her belly is the warm, dark sanctuary within. So call on Baubo to let your body and your laughter define your sacred and sexual space. She's a fine companion to have at your side through your child-birthing, child-rearing years and beyond.

9

BEYOND MONOGAMY

Affairs and Other Dynamics That Go Bump in the Night

AFFAIR! The word can strike like a stake through the heart. When sexual relationships burst the boundaries mapped out by culture, there's no more sex-as-usual. Your desire either plummets or it balloons bigger than life. The earth moves, the seas part, lightning hits. As a British colleague puts it, "An affair can play silly buggers with our sexual energy." This isn't just folklore turned pop psych. As I've reported earlier, brain studies on love and rejection show a picture of our neurotransmitters gone berserk.

Marry and remain faithful until death: this is sexual advice we were all given as children. But in today's complex society we aren't all able—or willing—to toe this marital line. Census figures show that married-couple households are now a minority in America. And surveys reveal that having more than one intimate partner is the norm in some 85 percent of cultures around the globe. Our own sky-high rates of infidelity, divorce, and single-parent families suggest that a just-say-no injunction isn't keeping all of us locked into relationships that aren't working. Four in five women who answered the ISIS survey say that commitment with their partners is what makes sex most satisfying—but that sexual commitment isn't always with their husbands. In fact, sex is *least* satisfying with their husbands say almost one in six of them, and over one in thirty say they find sex to be most satisfying during affairs outside of marriage.

The truth is, a wide discrepancy sometimes exists between the domestic and the erotic, as therapist Esther Perel points out in *Mating in Captivity*. So for a full understanding of the issues involved in sexual desire, it's important to factor in some of our struggles with sexual commitment: monogamy, affairs, and open relationships, for they all affect our sexual desire—the highs, the lows, and at least some of the in-betweens.

When He *Has the Affair*

There's far more permission in this culture for men to engage in affairs than there is for women—what else is new? An estimated 70 percent of married men have "cheated" on their wives—*cheat* is the unforgiving term that expresses the effect of secret-keeping and lack of trust. When this happens, women can feel devastated—betrayed, hurt, and filled with self-blame. I've heard woman after woman blurt forth her fear that she wasn't attractive enough, sexy enough, *woman* enough to keep her husband satisfied and at home, nose to the marital grindstone.

I can empathize. I've been through it, too. For me it was an emotional roller-coaster trying to seduce him back into the marriage—along with fantasies of suicide, murder, and wouldn't it just serve his extracurricular sweetie right if I planted a bomb in her pink suburban mailbox. In my less-manic periods I felt breach of promise, lack of agency, and for months so much shame I couldn't share my feelings with anyone who could help. As is true for countless other couples, that affair was emblematic of marital baggage that was already bogging down the relationship—and was the straw that finally broke it.

The good news is that I ultimately gained resilience and perspective, which helped me open my heart for other women undergoing their own versions of the cheating game. And I'm now living proof that it's possible to move beyond hurt and rage and pain to reclaim your sexual desire—and your life.

Fallout from your partner's affair

In my therapy work I've seen affairs set off a landslide of mistrust and rage—and this is true for lesbian partners as well as heterosexual ones. Some couples are able to dig their way back to the surface, and some are not. I've learned that the pain that works its way to the heart's core is often not solely about the sexual infidelity. It's about emotional and spiritual disconnection. It's about the shock of realizing the person you thought was your intimate is now a stranger. It's about the betrayal of cultural expectations, too. We spend our girlhoods hearing people we trust tell us, "faithful is good" and "unfaithful is bad." But we haven't been taught to think about these phrases with any complexity.

What does "faithful" actually mean? Faithful to whom? To what? What exactly *were* our vows to each other—and how do they translate to our lives today? How do they affect our sexual desire? What are our responsibilities to ourselves, our partners—and our children? Do we teach our kids through what we say or through what we do? For some women the ongoing agony is that they failed to speak up for what they wanted and needed—often (and this is the saddest part) because they didn't *know* what they wanted or needed.

Sometimes rage and outrage are warranted. You may need to stamp and scream to mobilize these energies and let your partner know the depth of your feeling. Other times you might do well to take a compassionate approach—understanding that your partner's affair isn't so much a reflection of you as it is of your partner, *his* desires, *his* personal path. In most cases, your partner isn't trying to mess up your life by engaging in an affair. Rather, he's simply trying to find a way to be happy. Still, openhearted detachment is tough to come by when you're plucking another woman's hairs off his sports jacket and examining his shirt collars for her lipstick. Or, as one client did, finding a credit card printout of the pricey restaurants he frequented with a gay male lover.

An emergency room nurse relates how her husband's affair plunged her into relational chaos, rupturing their spiritual connection as well as their sexual connection.

> I hated him at the moment, but yet I loved him so deeply—the pain was so deep. Weeks went by. I said things to hurt him and distanced myself from him in conversation and touch. When I came to terms with the situation and could forgive him, the first night we made love was so intense. We made total eye contact. No words were said, and I cried. The release of tension was wonderful.

It seems that trust might have begun to regenerate at this point except for his attitude about her looks—an attitude seemingly dictated by media stereotypes and a dominator mind-set that separated his sexual interest from any shred of empathy and caring. It was these that brought into vivid focus that he was not committed to marriage with her—body, mind, heart, and soul. Instead, he was caught up in an image of what he saw as female perfection. She felt she might as well have been a life-sized doll.

> The fact that I could forgive him was great, but I can't seem to put it completely behind me. He has made it a point that he loves big-breasted, slim blondes. Here I am, a small-breasted slim brunette. At times I feel that I must compete and can't. I can't totally trust him. Therefore at times sex turns me off.

The gist of her husband's message? "I want you to look sexy—but don't be too *sexual*. Just look good and lie still. Don't ask long-term commitments of me. And whatever you do, don't ask me to change my mind or feel any emotions." For a woman just summoning the courage to peek through her defensive armor, his response was destined to thrust her deeper into hiding—and deliver a potentially mortal wound to her sexual desire.

Her story raises an important point about body image and sexual desire, even beyond the complication of an affair. As social critic Susan Faludi writes in *Backlash,* women are expected to maintain "acceptable roles"— and look like movie stars (think "big-breasted, slim blondes"). But it's tough to invest in standards like these and also stay open to the multidimensional possibilities of sexual partnership and sacred union outlined elsewhere in this book. For these involve attitudes that look far beneath the skin and beyond it.

WHAT AN AFFAIR MAY MEAN FOR HIM

It's not that all men who have affairs are insensitive oafs incapable of complex loving. Too many men marry young, still in the grip of "real man" expectations. As outlined in the previous chapter, they may enter into their first long-term relationships without a clue as to how to express their sexual feelings, let alone how to connect with a partner or with a power beyond themselves. Sometimes the first stirring of whole-person awareness filters through from outside the marriage bond. When this occurs, a newly awakened man can become enchanted. Former promises and commitments can seem far away.

"Spiritual sex took me by surprise," admits a physician who'd been in a "functional but sterile" marriage for ten years, which he said counseling hadn't helped. Then he fell in love with a colleague.

> When it finally became sexual, it shook us ... Neither of us had ever heard of "spiritual sex" nor had there been any attempt to produce that. There was simply a deep, deep desire in each of us to give all we had to give to the other in response to the deep understanding and acceptance we had experienced from the other. What resulted was so profound that it left both of us weeping. We were overwhelmed with gratitude to each other for the healing that it brought. We were in awe of and overwhelmed with gratitude to a Creator who had made something so exquisite. We finally knew, without having to say it, what Scripture means when it says, "the two shall become one flesh." And so our sexual relationship remained in the few months that we shared it.

This man did not throw over his marriage. He and his new love agreed to stop meeting. But neither did he ever fully recover from the power of his affair. He says he used the experience as a powerful teaching to help right his sinking marital ship. Having tasted the forbidden and "exquisite" joys of loving as "one flesh," he tried to become a more attentive, compassionate, and sexually satisfying husband.

> My wife and I have had extensive counseling and have made great progress in our marriage. We now have a tender, committed, loving relationship and sex is better than it used to be. But it is not anything like that which so totally took me by surprise.

Many men who answered the ISIS survey wrote movingly of their affairs—and many women, too. The bottom line: affairs can be complex for men as well as for women. While there may be plenty of men who are rotten low-down deadbeat dads who persist in conquests and escapes from emotional responsibility, there are also men who are genuinely seeking what so many women seek. That is, "something more." Of course we have the right to rage and recompense when we're left in the lurch. Yet as I listen closely to the stories some men tell me about the quality of their sexual affairs, I'm surprised and delighted to find them filled with heart and soul as well as temporary physical excitement.

When Women Have Affairs

I don't see much written about how extramarital affairs can be positive for women. Mostly the news is about infidelity, secrecy, addiction, dysfunction, pain, and immoral behavior. God forbid women should get to do what men have had permission to do since the dawn of time.

So one of the big surprises of the ISIS survey was the passion with which women wrote about the spiritual quality of sexual desire during their affairs. I'm not talking only about the responses of sexual liberals with fringe religious practices. Many women in traditional marriages and mainstream religions—Southern Baptists, Mormons, and Roman Catholics, among others—said they experienced the most meaningful sex of their lives in their affairs, not in their church-sanctified marriages. (These real-life stories remind me of the sudden opening of Francesca, the farmer's wife, when she encounters her photographer lover in the *Bridges of Madison County*—well, with Meryl Streep and Clint Eastwood playing the parts, what do you expect.)

I mention these women here not to advocate for extramarital activity, for I've already pointed out the heartache and disruption this can cause. Rather, I include these women to raise yet another curtain on the kinds of conditions that allow us to rediscover our wellsprings of sexual passion.

Women describe their affairs as: "spiritual and warm," "overwhelming and powerful," filled with "intense connection, long hours of touching, soul kissing, talking, laughing, and relishing one another." For some women, their affairs embody the thrill of letting themselves be "bad girls," outside society's rules. An empty-nester says she reveled in "the danger, the naughtiness of it . . . it feels wild and totally abandoned and fulfilling."

Even beyond the adrenaline rush of rule breaking, affairs help some women enjoy significant firsts. These include: first eye contact during sex, first "deeply intimate experience," and first intimations that sexuality and spirituality are inextricably connected. All of these act as powerful aphrodisiacs.

In terms of reviving flagging libido, it may seem that an affair can be just what the doctor ordered. Or even better. A physician may prescribe testosterone, but as Helen Fisher's brain research shows, the new love and excitement of an affair may flood you with hormones that compel you to say "Yes."

WHAT PRICE AFFAIRS?
THE DISEASE, THE GUILT, THE MONEY . . .

Clearly, an affair can offer the potential for peak sexual experiences. But it's not that way for all women all the time. There can be a heavy price to pay for this route to sexual excitement. First, there's physical danger. Not only is your whole life complicated by an affair, there can be specific physical risks. We live in an age of HIV/AIDS, herpes, chlamydia, and other sexually transmitted horrors that don't rear their heads in romantic movies like *The Bridges of Madison County*. So it's crucial for you to know that when you have sexual intercourse, you are, in effect, having intercourse with every partner your partner has ever had intercourse with. If you do the math, you can understand how crucial it is for you to use condoms to protect yourself and your unwary partners—and to open up responsible communication with all the partners involved, if that is possible.

To find more information on preventing sexually transmitted infections, there are countless websites devoted to safe sex, and I urge you to research them if either you or your partner is engaging in sexual intercourse with other partners—or if you suspect this may be the situation. Better still, your local AIDS action program or Planned Parenthood may have counselors who can advise you in the practical ways of safer sex.

Aside from the potential for disease, affairs offer other sources of angst. Some women can't stand the strain of living a double life. Sometimes there's disillusionment. After the first flush of lust some women find themselves in yet another rotten relationship—one woman says she ended up feeling like "just another notch in his headboard." And even the most compelling affairs can be fraught with just too much complexity and drama. The anguish of choosing between husband and extramarital "soulmate" is an ongoing theme for women. The intensity of passion flung one woman squarely onto the horns of her basic conflicts: should she be loyal to her marriage—or should she follow her longings of body, heart, and soul? Both options led her through agonizing paths.

> I am very much in love with my lover, but truly love my husband deeply and don't believe in breaking up the marriage. However, only my soulmate (lover) has been able to fully tap into my spirituality as a woman and make the soul connection.

And then there's the guilt. Another woman wrestles with how to maintain long-term commitments both in her marriage and beyond.

> Sex was always purely physical with my husband. He placed guilt on me when I did not exhibit the sexual drive that he did. When I met my other partner, sex took on a new meaning, but guilt for "cheating" often took over.

Despite the double dose of guilt this woman describes, there were rewards that kept her in this affair for twenty-one years and still counting.

> He completely accepts me at a very high spiritual level. Meanwhile I have always been committed to my marriage, though attempts to raise the physical to the spiritual have exploded in my face.

And then there's violence. The woman above doesn't explain what her marital "explosions" are. But my clinical experience has taught me that too many men in this culture are socialized from boyhood to believe they're Top Banana. Many men evolve beyond this conditioning—they learn to listen, feel, and become true partners. But those who stay mired in dominator mode tend to take automatic charge of the checkbook, the car, and also the sexual rituals. They can feel backed into a scary corner when they're asked to deliver emotional understanding and spiritual affirmation, because they've never learned to excel in these spheres of relationship.

Scared men often plead cluelessness—because God forbid they should acknowledge their fear; that would blow their "real man" image. Or they erupt with anger. During a therapy session, a client's husband yelled, "Pull your goddamn self together!" when she asked him for a hug. Other times, a man who is scared will plunge himself into overwork or affairs—finding a new project or new woman to master.

As a sex therapist, I've witnessed countless variations on these explosive impasses. The good news is that they're not always inevitable. I've seen men soften their defenses when they learn it's possible to feel the full range of their emotions and still maintain a sense of integrity. I've seen them summon up the courage to empathize—and for some men it does take enormous courage, because it's a brand-new behavior.

I've also seen women give up whining when they feel their male partners soften. I've seen them find persuasive language, and body language, to ask for what they want—another act of enormous courage. For a woman who's been conditioned to say only "Yes, dear," it can be a life-changing event for her to straighten her spine and speak clearly in her own behalf. It's thrilling when these shifts happen, and it's one of the reasons I cherish my work.

Then there are the survival issues—money and safety and self-esteem. A minimum-wage gardener speaks of juggling the complexities involved in her decision to leave her husband, so "my soulmate and I will be together for the rest of our lives." On the one hand, she's determined to become self-sufficient before she leaves so she won't enter into yet another dependent relationship:

> I'm trying to get into a good job with a future, and until I do that I can't leave—even though he begs me all the time to leave my husband and move in with him. I can't or won't do that. I have to leave my husband on my own two feet, standing tall.

On the other hand, she fears that once she actually leaves her husband, the world will view her as a bad person.

> I'm sure you think I'm a bitch—I never thought anything like this would ever happen to me and I can't and I won't let the love of my life, my soul and spiritual mate, go.

Being branded as a bitch (or slut, or unprintable body part) is an archetypal fear for women. Our very survival has often depended on how others view us as nurturers, caretakers, and all-around ministering angels. Age-old punishments for women who break the sexual rules include burning, stoning, and shunning—ostracism from the village. We dread being stamped as the local Hester Prynne, sentenced to wear a proverbial scarlet "A" for "adulteress," for this can seem like a fate that is literally worse than death.

Then there are the religious taboos. Although in my ISIS survey, a number of devout women reported high-flying desire in their extramarital relationships, they also reported high-flying angst and confusion. A once-devout Mormon blames herself, not the rigidities of church morality. But in the end she stands firm for pleasure, refusing to recant her sexual freedom.

> I had sex for the first time when I was seventeen, ended up pregnant, and have been married for seven years. I have never enjoyed sex. I've always thought of it more as a chore than an enjoyable thing, until recently. I have been having an affair for a little over three months, and with him I love everything there is about sex and I truly feel it is a spiritual thing. I know that sounds stupid since affairs are religiously wrong, but there is no other way to explain what I experience when I am with him.

But many women knuckle under to church and culture, even though it hurts. Another woman expresses the other side of anguish. Having tasted what she calls the "holiness of pleasure" outside her marriage, she feels compelled to see herself as a sinner. She starts by describing what Saturday nights were like in her marriage—to a man trained in the homing-site model of sex.

> Sex with my husband is just that—sex! When he's in the mood he acts like a kid in a candy store—he reaches for my breasts

or his hands go straight between my legs. I try to tell him that there are other parts to me, but this is laughed at. Being married, I felt that this was how it was supposed to be (considering also that I didn't have too many other experiences). Also being abused as a child, having only those private areas touched, what else could I think?

When she meets the man with whom she's able to connect sex spiritually, a different story unfolds.

He left virtually no part of me untouched from my eyelids to my toes. It wasn't just the sex—it was the connection we felt. He felt it too. For the first time in my life I felt I could completely let go of stress and tension. My mind was clear, at peace, I felt so relaxed. When I was near him, I felt any problems weren't so bad.

Yet these lovers finally broke up in deference to their religious belief systems: "because I'm married and having an affair is a sin." Besides, who would stand up for her? According to church dogma, her actions were evil. An evangelical Christian elaborates on this view:

If I tried to explain the spirituality of the sex that I experienced they would tell me I was from the devil because "we don't believe in having affairs, and certainly any experience that came from an affair could not be considered spiritual."

The bottom line is that for some women affairs open them to new and extraordinary sexual landscapes. But to benefit from this influx of sexual energy, women may need to begin with a strong sense of self-esteem and an equally strong sense of belonging in their community. For both religion and culture malign women who engage in affairs. Affairs also carry with them a load of relational baggage, as outlined above. Still, we're not all born monogamous—which is a lifestyle dictated by religion and culture and not solely by our genetics. There are women for whom one partner is simply not enough. Clearly for some the desire for more than one partner becomes an untenable situation that dooms them to lives of misery. Other women have found a contemporary option—to enter into extracurricular relationships and invite their original partners to come, too. That option is called open marriage, or polyamory.

Polyamory
Beyond Affairs and Cheating

Polyamory literally means "loving many"—that is, maintaining intimate relationships with more than one partner at the same time. "Poly" relationships are different from affairs in that they're open—with information and agreement among all partners. That means no secrecy, no cheating, no excuses about late nights at the office, no hiding the phone bill, and ideally no ongoing guilt or jealousy. Sometimes the intimate relationships are not physically sexual. As the saying goes among aficionados—with affairs you get sex, with polyamory you get breakfast.

Polyamory represents the millennial evolution of the "open marriage" or "alternative lifestyle" movement that's been part of the American scene since the 1960s and before—through activities such as wife swapping, love-ins, swinging, and spinning the bottle. I'm not advocating polyamory as the lifestyle that's right for *you*. But for some women and men it fills a relational hunger as well as a desire for sexual adventure, says psychologist Deborah Anapol, author of *Polyamory,* a book that's helped define this lifestyle since the 1990s.

I first learned about the intricacies of open relationships from my friend and mentor James Ramey, who wrote a classic on this subject in the 1970s. His book *Intimate Friendships* addresses how multiple relationships can ramp up the sexual energy between the original committed partners as well as a variety of new "intimate friends." Intimate friendships can be exciting. They can be stereotype-busting. You can undergo a wholesale change of belief about what's right and normal. You can discover new depths of your own relationship expectations. It may occur to you for the first time that one person cannot fill all your partnership desires and needs. Simple as this idea sounds, it can be life-changing—and your libido can skyrocket.

You can also become overwhelmed. If you, or your partner, or both of you, enter into a sexual relationship with someone else, a thousand feelings can swirl—even when you wholeheartedly agree with the arrangement. You can feel elated, anxious, hurt, jealous, magnanimous, and more.

Whatever your response, it takes an enormous amount of time and energy to live fully in one successful intimate relationship, let alone two or three or more—especially if you have to keep your lifestyle hidden from your button-down boss or your buttoned-up father-in-law. Besides, when you open your relationship to other sexual partners, you and your original beloved are likely to require a good deal of extra focus on one another to keep your own bond strong and vital. That takes resilient hearts and constant communication. All of which become an opportunity for growth—and part of the process Ramey calls "peer bonding" as distinct from "pair bonding."

Some couples invite other couples to join in their sexual play. But polyamory depends on much more relational responsibility and consensuality than swinging, bottle spinning, and wife swapping. A seventy-four-year-old woman who's taken part in all these movements speaks of the need for "respect for all of our ideas, moods, and preferences."

> To enjoy oneness with others is a step I would like to see happen in our new millennium. I am not talking about promiscuity, rather a careful and responsible selection of couples, loving together with everyone's consent.

Another way to express "poly" is to invite a third "significant other" to share your whole relationship—literally join the family. A mediator with considerable relationship skills writes of a vibrant life she shares with both her husband and a younger man: "Mel walked into my joyful journey and took me further along the path of spirituality and sexuality." She says the intensity of their sexual experiences was mind-boggling. An interesting aspect of her story is that she and her husband consider him part of their family—and their relationships are fully accepted by all of their close friends and grown children.

> I am still very much in love with my husband of thirty-five years, who has been a constant companion on my spiritual and sexual journey in different ways than Mel. And Mel and I are still committed partners after more than five years. The three of us have become "co-creators" in our spiritual path together.

As the braiding of their relationships grew more intricate and vital, she says it became clear how each of these men fills a different role in her life—and in each other's. The rewards for the men include sexual intimacy with her—and also deep friendship with one another. The rewards for her are two devoted lovers—though she says she also revels in her days off, when she can kick back and enjoy some downtime.

The truth is that there is no one all-abiding blueprint for commitment that fits all sexual relationships—whether within the context of a conventional pair bond or outside it. Whatever your choices may be, it's crucial that you pay attention to your feelings and the feelings of your partner or partners, and adapt to circumstances as you go along. Below are questions that have helped many of my clients find the paths that are right for them.

Exploring Your Sexual Desire
Using the ISIS Wheel to Explore Your Relationship Options

As a therapist, I've learned that questions can sometimes be as therapeutic as definitive answers—often more so. They can shake shake loose stagnant patterns, open up new vistas, and suggest new solutions without dictating them. The intent of the questions below is not to say you ought to change your mind about a sexual lifestyle that you truly value, whether that's monogamy or any of the variations beyond monogamy. The intent is to encourage you to articulate what kinds of relationships move your life—and especially your sexual desire. Have a look at the questions and decide whether asking them might deepen and vitalize your sexual understanding about what you want. Then see if it feels right to ask them with your partner and discuss your answers with each other.

If you are being sexual with more than one partner, by all means share these questions with each of them. Or gather a trustworthy group of friends together and share them with the whole gang. Positive feedback can be an aphrodisiac. And negative feedback may not turn you on, but in the long run it can offer much food for thought.

Be sure to leave yourself plenty of time to process your feelings, as you're treading in potentially deep waters. These questions are not intended as a substitute for skilled therapy if that's what your situation warrants. The Resources section at the end of this book will guide you to finding a trained therapist in your area, and also, if you wish, to channels for opening your relationship and exploring polyamory with both pleasure and responsibility.

Exploring your physical path
What does your body tell you about your relationship choices?

Your body is infinitely intelligent, and if you listen closely to it, you'll learn much about how you respond to the relationship choices you're making—or that you feel are being made without your consent. Remember how I began this chapter: "Affair! The word can strike like a stake through the heart." The truth is, your thoughts and feelings can manifest in a startlingly physical way—and tapping into that information can help you know whether or not you're on the life path that's right for you.

You may be holding your thoughts and emotions in specific places. Perhaps you're knotting your brow in confusion, clenching your fists in anger, or hunching your shoulders in defeat—the list goes on. Conversely, you may feel like leaping for joy—opening your heart in love, sighing with pleasure. Spend some quiet time checking in with your body and you can probably come up with many more places that are expressing the tension or release you feel in your relationships.

> As you sit quietly and breathe into these places in your body, what can you feel? Begin with your face, your hands, your feet, your jaw. How about your neck, your diaphragm, your buttocks, your genitals?
>
> When you think about marriage, affairs, or poly relationships what do you notice happening in these places—are they tensing or releasing?

If you change your breathing or your body posture does this change your thoughts and feelings?

EXPLORING YOUR EMOTIONAL PATH
WHAT ARE YOU AFRAID OF LOSING? ARE YOU JEALOUS?

There may be much to lose when you step outside the relationship boundaries set by society—or even when you think outside those boundaries. Rewards for staying in a conventional marriage include economic stability, a resident sexual partner, a life companion, and a co-parent for your children—no small compensations. Some women fear losing these when their mates have affairs. Some fear losing these when they enter into affairs or poly relationships themselves. Others fear losing these even when they're fully ensconced in a monogamous relationship. These fears constrict the flow of desire.

What aspects of relationship do you fear you can't live without?

What might your life look like without these?

How do you feel as you picture yourself without these?

Fear of loss can create jealousy. What is the color of your jealousy? What color is your love? Your pain? Your commitment? Your trust? Your need? Get out the magic markers and start drawing pictures if you like. I borrowed this exercise from my colleagues Leah Kliger and Deborah Nedelman, authors of *Still Sexy after All These Years*—who traveled around the country asking groups of older women to describe the color of their sexual feelings. Sometimes using a mode other than talking can help you express the inexpressible. Your heart may feel lighter after you do this exercise—as long as you understand it's not an art contest.

EXPLORING YOUR MENTAL PATH
WHAT DO YOU BELIEVE ARE YOUR RELATIONSHIP OBLIGATIONS?

Most of us were raised to think that marriage is the only responsible context for sexual intimacy and that sex outside of marriage is immoral. Yet most relationships today are not lifelong. And brain research suggests that human beings are not necessarily hardwired for monogamous relationships.

Who is voicing the morality message in your life now? Your religion? Your neighbor? Your parents? Your grown children? You?

This isn't a pitch for you to go against the grain of your true beliefs. But years of listening to clients has taught me that sometimes our beliefs aren't really *ours*. They may belong to somebody else, and we've taken them on out of a desire to be good, to please others, to be loved and accepted. If that's the case, it may be time for you to update your beliefs—or to reaffirm the ones you really do hold dear. This is an opportunity to make sure that your moral convictions about sexual relationship really are *your* dream, not somebody else's dream for you. So ask yourself the questions below. Listen to your answers, and share them with your partner or partners.

> What are your criteria for a happy, healthy, loving sexual relationship?
>
> What are your personal ground rules for relaxation, freedom, and sexual excitement?
>
> What are your sexual obligations to your partner?
>
> What are your obligations to your family in terms of how you express your sexuality? (This means parents, children—whoever may be affected by your actions.)
>
> What are your obligations to yourself?

Hint: Think about time. Think about honesty. Think about listening, respect, attention—all the elements of desire that women talk about throughout this book. This is your chance to explore what you want in your life right now.

EXPLORING YOUR SPIRITUAL PATH
WHAT TRUTHS DO YOU WANT YOUR PARTNER TO KNOW ABOUT YOUR RELATIONSHIP OPTIONS?
Here's an opportunity for a conversation with your partner—in which you allow yourself to reveal your deepest feelings and convictions about your

sexual relationship together and how you experience your sexual desire and your commitment to your partner's sexual well-being.

Set aside at least a couple of hours of protected time and space. Turn off your phone and any other interruptions. Make sure you're comfortable.

Ask your partner to lie down, eyes closed. Hunker down next to him or her.

Speak your heart—with urgency—as if your partner has less than an hour to live. What are the very last words you want your partner to hear from you—about desire, about life, about love, about the meaning of your relationship? This simple exercise can be a powerful reminder of what is really important.

If you're stumped on how to begin, tell the story of how you met and what drew you together in the first place. Sometimes telling an old story puts a new story in perspective. If your relationship is vital and full of zest, talking about your early attractions can reinforce your sexual attraction toward each other now. If it's shaky, going back to basics may shift the energy between you so that you can remember what's good and sexy about your relationship—or at least what was good and sexy. If you can't find anything good or sexy to say about your relationship in the present, that is a painful truth. But perhaps it needs to be said—and this is your chance to allow that truth to emerge.

When you've spoken your heart, then reverse your roles. Now it's your turn to hear the "last words" your partner wants you to hear.

To complete the exercise, both of you get to return miraculously to life! Make eye contact, make heart contact, make physical contact—and tell each other what you believe is the heart and soul of your life, separately and together. Now that you have set the scene for such open sharing, this is a prime opportunity for you to discuss all aspects of your sexual desire—the depths of your commitment to each other, and perhaps exploring other sexual relationships. Take this chance to reach beyond your usual comfort zone. Allow your dreams to surface. If those dreams include sexual partners beyond your present relationship, let your heart determine whether or not to speak of them at this moment—and what words to use. This is a moment you can use to voice your appreciation for your partner and the relationship. Say what you have loved about each other. Say what you have learned by being together. Allow this part to go on for a long time if you like. See what unfolds between you.

10

LIVING CURLY IN A STRAIGHT CULTURE
When Desire Meets Sexual Orientation

As you've seen in earlier chapters, sexual desire can plummet with life changes created by childbirth, affairs, and losing yourself in your partner—to name a few of the big ones. Now let's explore another crucial piece of the desire picture: the nuances of your sexual orientation. Who have you been most drawn to over your lifetime? Is it men? Is it women? Is it both? Are you sure? Though it can be scary to begin to ask yourself these questions, it's important to know the answers. Otherwise you might wake up one morning and find you're in bed with the wrong partner.

When we explore the intricacies of sexual desire—what we want, how it feels, and what it means in our lives—there's not always a solid line between straight and gay. Years of listening to women have shown me just how wavy that line can be. When you look at the full range of your own sexual longings and how they fit with your choice of partner, you may find some gray areas. This may be true even if you think you're totally one orientation or totally the other.

Though most of us are heterosexual, the widely accepted figure is that somewhere between 4 and 10 percent of contemporary Americans are lesbian or gay—the national census doesn't count bisexuals. Fourteen percent of ISIS survey respondents reported that they were lesbian, gay, or bisexual. These figures may or may not be meaningful, though, because it's tough to gather accurate statistics on sexual orientation. For one thing, sexual desire may be fluid over the course of our lives. Some women have a lifelong attraction to men. Some women knew they loved women from the moment they wrestled little Suzie to the grass during first-grade recess. But other women aren't so sure over the long term. Maybe they felt—and behaved—entirely heterosexual until their forties or fifties, when they suddenly found themselves in love again, this time with a woman. The fluidity of sexual orientation can work the other way, too—from lesbian to heterosexual. Some of today's savvy college students flow with the shifting sands of sexual orientation. They refer to themselves as LUGs—Lesbian Until Graduation.

To further complicate the gathering of numbers, there's the social stigma of being "different," and the all-too-tangible risks—which range from job loss to hate crimes. Surely these prevent some survey respondents from identifying themselves as anything but heterosexual. Playwright Oscar Wilde, who was imprisoned in 1890s England for "gross indecency" (he was flagrantly gay), famously called homosexuality "the love that dares not speak its name." Even though right now in America we can't be thrown in jail for being lesbian or gay, we can have problems renting an apartment; we can lose custody of our children; we can be denied access to a dying partner. So sexual relationships that brand us as different are not always a bed of roses, and women often choose to stay in conventional marriages even if they are attracted to other women. As a client once aptly put it, "It's not easy living a curly life in a straight culture."

In the mid-twentieth century, sex researcher Alfred Kinsey addressed the mutable nature of sexual orientation when he became the first to place heterosexuality and homosexuality on a continuum—using a zero-to-six scale. *Zero* means you lust only after partners of the opposite sex, and *six* means you lust only after same-sex partners. Most of us fall somewhere between, said Kinsey.

Charting Yourself from Straight to Curly
Your Behaviors, Fantasies, and Desires

Are you heterosexual, lesbian, or fluctuating somewhere between? You can chart your own history of partner choice on the Kinsey scale, which ranks your desires and fantasies, as well as your actual behaviors. Where do you place yourself between the two poles: zero (totally heterosexual) and six (totally lesbian)? Try applying this scale to various periods in your life and see what you notice. Where were you in high school—or even before? Where were you in your twenties, thirties, forties, and beyond?

Who were you sexual with? Who did you lust after? Who turned you off? And most important, where do you place yourself on this scale right now?

The Kinsey Scale of Sexual Orientation
Creatively Adapted for Women's Relationships

From Alfred Kinsey, et al. *Sexual Behavior in the Human Male* (Philadelphia: W.B. Saunders, 1948).

0   Exclusively heterosexual—you're straight as an arrow, you only have eyes for men

1   Predominantly hetero but you may perk up when a woman walks by

2   Predominantly hetero but women definitely interest you

3   You're happy to swing either way

4   Predominantly lesbian but men definitely interest you

5   Predominantly lesbian but you may perk up when a man walks by

6   Exclusively lesbian—you're definitely curly, you only have eyes for women

---

Despite the possible difficulties, sexual desire sometimes blossoms most fully outside the cultural box. For some women it bursts into full flower with other women. This is what happened in my life. After two marriages to men, I suddenly looked at the woman who was my best friend and it dawned on both of us that we were deeply attracted to one another and destined to be much more than just friends.

That was twenty-seven years ago, and we've been committed life partners ever since. Yes, it was complicated. And of course there were others to consider—especially our then-teenage children. The details of how we worked it out could fill another book. Suffice it to say that we felt our relationship was remarkable then, we continue to feel that way, and we thank the universe every day that we are together. Truly for me, stepping into the relationship with her felt as if I'd reclaimed an unacknowledged half of my life. But what's also remarkable is that while I was with each of my two husbands (and we're talking a sum of seventeen years) I felt totally attracted to them. What broke up those relationships were personal conflicts, not sexual orientation, and I had no inkling that I would end up in partnership with a woman.

Maybe the no-inkling part was denial born of my tight-lipped WASP upbringing. Maybe it was born of the Western culture we live in. Women are not supposed to lust after other women, let alone enjoy long, deeply erotic partnerships with each other. This is a moral mandate with a long history, and sometimes the fact of women loving women is quite literally invisible. Queen Victoria (for one) is said to have declared, "Two women do such a thing? Never!" This kind of denial exists even today, even in the United States. Unless you live in a liberal community, lesbians may not even be talked about as real people—despite the TV outings of Ellen DeGeneres and Rosie O'Donnell. There may not even be a name for relationships that exist outside of heterosexual marriage. A longtime lesbian couple I know overheard a neighbor referring to them as "the *Lesbanians* who live next door."

Cultural dismissal can chip away at sexual desire. I know from personal experience how women can internalize this negativity. Guilt and shame may take over the place of healthy lust. When you're forced to hide your feelings, you're also holding back your flow of desire. If you want to maintain sexual energy and interest over your lifetime, you can't always "just say no" to sexual responses that don't fit society's idea of what you're supposed to feel toward whom.

What If You're Heterosexual—But Wondering?

I'm not suggesting that you leap into action every time you feel a sexual urge. But if you want to understand the full scope of your sexual desire—or lack of desire—I am urging you to summon the courage to be clear with yourself about your sources of sexual attraction. If you're in an intimate relationship with a man, and you find yourself drawn to a woman, you need to know that about yourself—whether or not you decide to act on this knowledge.

One of my watershed lessons as a sex therapist burst upon me during a session long ago with the third couple I ever saw—a man and woman whose presenting problem was her low desire. I couldn't seem to get a handle on why these two compatible and energetic people were having problems in bed, so I asked to see each one of them separately, hoping that might shake loose some helpful information. It was then that she confided she was madly in love and lust with the woman next door. Even though this predated my own epiphany of love and lust, I could see that here was trouble in paradise, indeed. Her disclosure rang in my brain with the clarity of trumpets. Ta da! You can't be sexually hot for your husband if you're really in love with a woman!

I've since learned to temper this categorical stance. I've met bisexual and polyamorous lovers who can maintain prodigious amounts of sexual energy for multiple partners—you met some of them in the previous chapter. But generally, it's been my clinical experience that desire doesn't flourish equally in two places at once. If you're trying to re-vamp desire with a man, and your sexual attentions are focused on a woman, you can bolster yourself with the latest hormone therapy and you can work every technique in the sex therapy manuals, but chances are you'll still end up saying a resounding "Not tonight, dear."

Therapy sessions with this couple turned out not to be about helping them rebalance the desire discrepancies that brought them to my office. Instead, the focus was on supporting them both in dissolving their marriage as gracefully as possible as she moved inexorably toward a full-time partnership with the woman of her desire. And these sessions generated for me a great deal of thinking about sexual orientation and how it affects sexual desire—for women and men, separately and together.

Woman Plus Woman—Mirrors of Body and Soul

Women who love women often speak of being attracted to the pleasures of touching someone "built like me"—the physical presence and energy, the hair, the smell, the softness. One lesbian woman who answered the ISIS survey says, "From our first kiss, our first touch . . . she knew me inside and out. I never dreamed of feeling that way emotionally and physically." Others speak of eye contact, of crying with the joy of feeling flesh on flesh, of "touching quietly and lightly—every touch was divine and orgasmic on every part of my body."

For some women, discovering that they are attracted to other women leads to a blossoming of desire, with new heights of pleasure and meaning. An engineer puts it this way:

> Not until I was with a woman did I know my own spiritual and sexual capacity. The joy of seeing another beautiful female body—the feel of her soft, smooth skin on mine—these things intensify the ecstasy of the sexual act, and the orgasms are truly moments of worship and reverence for the wondrous creator, whoever it may be.

A seventy-four-year-old author states emphatically, "In my years of sex with men, I never felt a spiritual component in sex. It was with another woman lover I first felt the spirituality of sex—being in love, that we were enveloped by love." A food service manager describes her "soulful" lesbian relationship as feeling totally unlike her five-year marriage to a man. During this marriage, she says, "the sex was awful. I did everything I could to not have sex. I even had an affair—it was an exciting thing for me—until we actually had sex. It too was horrible."

Some lesbians say their women lovers evoke more respect, empathy, sharing, and caring than their male partners. The women seem to recognize each other as more than just lovers—they're sister travelers on this planet. "Not that being with a woman is better or worse than a male, just different," explains a paralegal who describes herself as "a twenty-three-year-old female with an active sexual spirit." But she goes on to say that for her sex is in fact "better" with a woman. "If there is anything more spiritually fulfilling than the touch of a female I have not found it."

Another speaks of "erotic experiences that had sexual subtleties. It is possible to experience an orgasm without physical contact—and almost as good—you get to do it in public." (For more information on spontaneous orgasm see chapter 5 of *Women Who Love Sex*. It's a fascinating phenomenon that requires no touch, just an active imagination. One woman calls it "thinking off.")

For some women who love women, the mirroring of each other's bodies leads to a mirroring of souls—which may mean transcending some of the boundaries and realities that keep us tied to the earth plane. A teacher describes an adventure that took place when she was newly in love.

> I experienced an orgasm so explosive that I felt I had completely disintegrated as "myself" and became one with the entire cosmic flow of energy, a ribbon of light in a vast and unending dance. I felt united not with my partner but with God.

A physical therapist also looks back to describe cosmic orgasms with her women partners.

> My first continuous orgasm was so powerful and with such a powerful, focused woman lover that my awareness lifted beyond the usual body pleasure into a timeless sense of beingness and oneness with cosmic energy . . . Another was when I felt that we both were rising into the stratosphere together connected by a silver cord.

These experiences follow a pattern I describe in *The Heart and Soul of Sex*—a sense of traveling in time and space when physical, emotional, mental, and spiritual experience meet. Although the last two women mentioned using pot as part of their sexual adventures, thousands of women of all sexual orientations affirm that it's possible to reach this state of oneness without drugs or alcohol. Boundaries fade. Lifetimes merge. Desire and ecstasy are one. You become lighter, more open and expansive. You align with rainbows, sunsets, ocean, universe. You experience meetings and matings in other lifetimes. Magic is afoot.

"LESBIAN BED DEATH"

But life and love among women is not all magic. It's a sobering fact that many lesbians face denial, social stigma, and gay bashing, which is a well-documented fact of the American scene. These can affect lesbians' ability to hold jobs, get housing, raise children. Less well documented is how these kinds of stresses can also affect libido, especially when added to the everyday stresses of ongoing life—lack of time and energy, not to mention codependency, affairs, and other relationship problems we've looked at earlier.

"Lesbian bed death" is a gloomy phrase popularized in the 1980s by feminist humorist Kate Clinton to describe how sexual activity can go south once two women snuggle into sharing a home and a life. This is one of the stereotypes circulated about lesbian relationships, along with the classic two-liner about the haste with which two women may rush into nesting behavior once they've connected:

"What does a lesbian bring on her second date?"

Answer: "A moving van."

In fact, desire in lesbian relationships is fully as complex as desire in relationships between women and men. And because there's no penis-vagina intercourse to use as a benchmark, it's more difficult for researchers to assess intensity of desire by the usual standard of "how many times did you do it last month." We have to ask about nongenital responses too—for some women, hugging, kissing, and overall touching are what it's all about. And if we also ask questions about emotions and meanings, we most often find that sexual desire and satisfaction for lesbian women involve the whole person, the whole relationship.

My colleague Suzanne Iasenza, who conducts a therapy practice for lesbian couples in New York City, predictably finds multiple issues contributing to sexual desire—"passion isn't connected only to genital contact." Researchers who have investigated lesbian sexual desire from holistic perspectives also find that lesbians want much more than genital contact. They don't want less sex than women who partner with men, but they may want it differently, says Margaret Nichols, director of the Institute for Personal Growth in New Jersey. The lesbians in her research sample of over one thousand women desired just as much physical stimulation as the heterosexual women did. "The lesbian bed death thing is bogus," she says.

The truth is, lesbian desire is complex, and may be complicated by social stresses. We can't find adequate answers when we ask questions geared to institutions that are typically supportive of heterosexual couples. A prime example is the institution of marriage.

Same-Sex Marriage
Does it Enhance Desire?

It doesn't take a rocket scientist to guess the answer to this question. Marriage enhances desire for some lesbian women and not for others. When gay marriage went legal, many lesbians whooped, hollered, and tied the knot. May 17, 2004, was a night to remember in Cambridge, Massachusetts, where I live. Horns tooted and bells rang all over town—almost as much noise as when the Red Sox won the World Series. Legal marriage meant adoption rights and health insurance as well as hearts, roses, and blessings from liberal pulpits. The scientific studies aren't out yet, but stories from some of the blushing brides say marriage has enriched their fabric of sexual desire by upgrading their self-esteem, partner confidence, and status in the material world. For others, well, there have been lesbian divorces too, but so far, not at the 50 percent rate reported for heterosexual marriages.

Not every lesbian in the universe signed up to marry, of course—including my partner and me. We figured we'd already been there, done that. Besides, we were happy living our lives without tying a civil knot. Marriage is not always a panacea, especially for women who'd had iffy marriages with men. In fact, generations of lesbians have already figured out how to settle into partnerships with all the earmarks of marital bliss—love, respect, shared goals, fluid roles, community support, nourishing sex—everything but financial and legal benefits and universal religious sanction.

Many of the traditional reasons for marrying are outdated, asserts Stephanie Coontz, director of public education for the Council on Contemporary Families and author of *Marriage, a History: How Love Conquered Marriage*. She writes that even in the heterosexual world, marriages based on love and intimacy have long supplanted marriages based on status and convenience—at least in Western culture, at least for the most part. She also argues that birth control and assisted reproduction have forever altered the procreative function of marriage.

What about raising children? Lesbian theologian Mary Hunt, co-director of the Women's Alliance for Theology, Ethics, and Ritual (WATER) agrees with Coontz that we don't need a legal marriage bond to be good parents—or good partners. What keeps the energy alive is not a legal bond. It's remaining conscious to your own needs and the needs of the relationship.

How Does Bisexuality Affect Desire?

In some respects, bisexual relationships may be even more counterculture than lesbian ones, says Loraine Hutchins, a coeditor of the classic anthology *Bi Any Other Name: Bisexual People Speak Out*. This, she points out, is because having both male and female lovers flies in the face of ideals about monogamy and commitment—the sacrosanct notion that we're supposed to stay sexually bound to one partner (preferably heterosexual) our whole lives long.

Woody Allen once quipped that being bisexual doubles your chance of getting a date on Saturday night. But bisexuality is more than a license to flirt pandemically at your local singles bar. It can be a direct path to the complex realm of sexual desire: body, mind, heart, and spirit. It involves your senses—both men and women can look good, smell good, feel good. It involves your energy, your magnetism, and your capacity for connection with your own femaleness and maleness—elements of our being that the visionary psychiatrist Carl Jung calls the *anima* and *animus* that inhabit all of us and invest us with the impulse to reach out for pleasure.

Many bisexual women say that what they want in sexual relationships goes way beyond physical kicks. "Just having sex got boring—even if it was fabulous sex—Tantric with forty-two orgasms a night," says a TV producer. "Something in me knew there was more and it was meant to be experienced deeper." This is the sense of "more" that so many women in my therapy practice say they yearn for in their search for sexual wholeness. It's a sense of total connection. A place where "thou shalt nots" and gender distinctions seem to melt like proverbial lemon drops.

"I prefer men but love women endlessly," says another bisexual woman. And another says, "I like to know my body and personality can affect men *and* women." Still another observes: "There is something extremely powerful in union, be it same sex or opposite sex union . . . each is an awe-inspiring experience."

As these women illustrate, a "bi" lifestyle ranges way beyond the Mars-Venus dichotomy outlined in chapter 7, which depends on a double standard of sexual desire—he wants sex, she wants love (and on and on). Instead, bisexual women say desire often hinges on a sense of equilibrium that is uniquely provided by their partnerships with both women and men—"the balance of yin-yang, male-female energies," says an art teacher. A customer service rep adds her own wisdom, which includes much more than just sex. "Being bi is about balance and growth, joy and pleasure, the things which guide us when times are dark, make life worth living when it's not."

It's this sense of sexual balance that allows for a full range of sexual desire, asserts a graphic artist—who says the first time she felt "complete" was when she and her husband invited another woman to make love with them. For her, this sexual blending of female and male was more than the physical pleasure, or the novelty, or the thrill of bending rules. It was a true wrinkle in time—as if she had stepped into a realm beyond her knowing. And the experience transformed her life.

> I felt whole, as if two halves had just come together. I felt loved and accepted for who I really was. I also had an epiphany of walking out into the universe and being one with all—being able to see far into my past and far into my future. And at the same time experiencing fully that exact moment.

Many women who answered my ISIS survey speak as if embracing their desire for both men and women is a kind of magical "coming out" to themselves. For some the route is physical—a path of lips and genitals, slithering hips, sweet breath, salty tongue, and other delicious sensations. Other women say it begins with heart-to-heart connection—sharing feelings, making eye contact. Or with a spiritual practice—a meditation, a prayer, a conversation with God that opens up a place of "mystery and acceptance."

The section that follows suggests some practices you can use to find your own place of sexual mystery and acceptance—to bring the energy of newness and wonder into your hearts and minds—whether your partners are women, men, or both.

Exploring Your Sexual Desire
Using the ISIS Wheel to Understand Your Sexual Orientation

Exploring your sexual orientation and identity can be complex, because sexual attraction may involve more than gay, straight, and something in between. A full exploration of all of the possibilities is beyond the scope of this book—but at least some of them deserve a mention here.

Perhaps your sexual journey has you traveling into the realm of transgender—transitioning into sexual reassignment, from male to female, for instance. Or perhaps you or your partners identify as "queer" or "questioning" your sexual status. Or maybe you're among the one in every two thousand adults who is born intersex—with ambiguous genitalia. Terminology for such distinctions is often expressed in initials—and sometimes makes me feel as if I'm swimming in alphabet soup. MTFHLGBIQQ—any activist sexologist can tell you these initials stand for male-to-female, heterosexual, lesbian, gay, bisexual, intersex, queer, and questioning. What they actually spell are the relational anomalies created by extremely complex and individual sexual lifestyles—and if any of them figure in your sexual framework, they can color how you experience desire.

However you identify, your most profound sexual turn-ons are likely to be emotional, spiritual, and mental as well as physical. This holds true for your partner choice as well. So whether you want to keep it simple or make it complex, here's an opportunity to locate who you're attracted to in terms of your physical sensations, your emotional feelings, your thoughts, and what sex means in your life. Think of it as: the Kinsey scale meets the ISIS Wheel. (The Kinsey scale that appears on page 133 is abbreviated below.)

THE KINSEY SCALE OF SEXUAL ORIENTATION

Exclusively straight 0 — 1 — 2 — 3 — 4 — 5 — 6 Exclusively lesbian

---

CHARTING YOUR PHYSICAL PATH
WAKING UP YOUR BODY

Let yourself focus on your breathing and other physical sensations as you remember the people in your life you've been sexually attracted to. Are they men or women—or both? Who do you feel in your bones is the fairest one of all? Whose smells and tastes are most tantalizing? Who puts wings on your heels? Who makes your heart thump with love? Who makes you juicy? Who do you want to make love with?

Conversely, have there been sexual partners in your life that you definitely did not want to make love with—and don't, ever? Is there anyone in your past or present that you want to run away from? Or who makes your throat close up? Or your skin crawl? Or turns your stomach?

As you rank your sexual wants and wishes on this scale of sexual orientation, what do your body responses tell you about whether you're straight or curly? If you listen closely to what your body says, you'll find enormous wisdom there. And you may uncover some surprising news about your sexual choices. You're not making value judgments. All you have to do is turn to the body channel and pay attention.

CHARTING YOUR EMOTIONAL PATH
OPENING UP YOUR CLOSET

Now chart your emotional attraction on the scale above. Ask yourself the same kinds of questions: Who do you open up to and who do you shrink from? Who do you laugh with and look forward to sharing yourself with? As you chart your life on the scale, you may find yourself uncovering other core issues about desire that you've found difficult to address before now. Maybe these issues are centered around love, self-image, trust, power, or vulnerability. Maybe they're around sticking to social convention, or moving beyond it. Maybe they're around reclaiming a part of your life that you never knew existed, or never dared let yourself know about. If this occurs for you, be assured that you're not alone—countless other women have felt this way—including me. If these are new feelings for you, be aware that some emotional turbulence may blow in.

Your most important lesson as you do these exercises may be to open your heart to the changes taking place in you. Our sexual desires are not fixed stars. They shift and move over the course of our lives. If you have any doubts about this, ask anyone in their sixties or seventies if they honestly want exactly the same things they wanted in their twenties. The changes in our desire may involve changing our choice of partner as well as how we want to use our sexual energy.

CHARTING YOUR MENTAL PATH
LETTING GO OF JUDGMENT

The choices you make about your sexual orientation may also show up as lessons on the mental path of the ISIS Wheel. This is the path of discernment, the place where you can evaluate society's messages about sex and how they affect your life. A big lesson here may involve suspending judgment about your own choice of partner. What's the big deal about same-sex relationships? And who is it a big deal for? You? Your parents? Your children? Your church? Your job?

This is an opportunity to chart your path again—this time in terms of the shoulds and oughts you learned about sexual orientation. Channeling your sexual desire onto a path it doesn't naturally want to go actually goes against the natural order. And I don't mean just people. Most vertebrates are heterosexual, assumedly to propagate the species. But scientists have found same-sex behavior across various species, from apes and dolphins to seagulls and, yes, penguins—despite all the family-values hoo-ha about the documentary film *The March of the Penguins.* For instance, in the winter of 2005 officials in Germany's Bremerhaven Zoo tried fruitlessly to separate three male penguin couples who refused to mate or even rub tummies with the female penguins in the zoo. If you're willing to have your perceptions really blown, read *Biological Exuberance* by Bruce Bagemihl, about homosexuality in the animal world, which investigates (in words I wish I'd thought of first) "the love that dares not bark its name."

CHARTING YOUR SPIRITUAL PATH
MOVING BEYOND TABOOS

Now chart yourself again on the zero-to-six scale, this time on the path of connection and meaning. It's from your spiritual path that you examine the significance of the sexual taboos you hold on to and how they relate to your life. Fear of being different can be a big one—and if you're sexually attracted to a woman, that definitely means "different" in the eyes of our culture, probably in the eyes of the religion you grew up in, as well. Fear always constricts the spirit—including your ability to reach out to others and even to define yourself. Here's a simple visualization to help you take the edge off your fear so you can determine your own sexual desires and behavior.

Whether you identify as lesbian, bi, or straight (or any other initials in the alphabet soup), I invite you look deeply inside yourself—to see what is right and true for you.

Imagine you have a magic mirror that allows you to see into your inner self. Look into this mirror now, and let yourself see reflected back to you the part of you that cares about women—the part who loves women and who feels an expanded sense of self in the presence of women—whether this expansion feels overtly sexual or not.

Take this woman-loving part of you by the hand and bring her to the edge of the ISIS Wheel. How do you see her entering into her sexual experience? Does she hang back at the perimeter or does she jump right into the center? Which paths does she take? Does she begin on the emotional path—where she opens her heart? Or the physical path—where she responds to the pulses of her body? Or the mental path—where she reevaluates the messages about her sexual desire? Or the spiritual path—where she weaves together the meanings of her sexual journey?

Look deeply into this mirror of yourself and honor her journey wherever it begins and wherever it takes her—and wherever it takes you. For her journey is your journey. Even where the path may be bumpy, it can lead you to reaffirm your own choice of partner—whether that's with a woman, a man, or both. Honoring the journey of this woman-loving part of you can also expand your present partnership possibilities, and help you respect the partnership choices of others.

When you're ready, thank this part of you for showing you her secrets of sexual desire. Bring yourself back to the here and now with a new sense of togetherness. A sense that you are a part of her life rather than apart from her life. A sense that you are able to make clear choices for yourself and that whatever your sexual choices are, you are not alone.

11

ABUSE AND TRAUMA
Exorcising Fear and Reclaiming Your Sexual Self

SEXUAL ABUSE AND TRAUMA cast a long shadow over our capacity for sexual desire. These can undermine our will to reach out to others, to connect with lust, love, or anything else that feels pleasurable and holy. I've heard countless survivors rage over their loss of innocence, loss of trust, loss of confidence, loss of joy and wholeness, loss of self. "I constantly felt unworthy and impure," says a journalist from Oregon. A New York editor calls the sense of loss "this hole in my heart," expressing the despair so many women bring into my practice. The agony can sometimes lie too deep for words, or even tears. And it can haunt us for life.

About a third of the women who answered my ISIS survey say they experienced sexual abuse as children, as adults, or as both. This corresponds with other national statistics on sexual abuse, though responsible numbers are notoriously difficult to come by because so much sexual abuse goes unreported. Also because there are so many degrees of sexual abuse—a drunken grope, a gang rape, beating, repeated torture—all these are obviously different, but they can fall under the same general category.

Painful sexual memories often date from childhood: recollections of our hands slapped, bound, or tied to the bedpost to prevent us finding the delicious little button between our legs. Murky scenes of Uncle Harry, or the babysitter, or Daddy who visited in the night and threatened we'd die if we ever told. The memories aren't always clear. A client struggled with the secrecy surrounding the midnight violations that had occurred for every female member of her family. They happened after everybody was asleep, so nobody could remember them or talk about them in the light of day. The bruises never showed. Did they really happen—or was it all a bad dream?

Abuse doesn't have to be directly sexual to thwart our capacity for sexual desire. Abuse might take the form of domestic violence—from physical assault and battering to more subtle methods of control. One woman talks about life with her ex-husband. "He called me 'fatso.' He wouldn't let my mother come to the house. He withheld everything from hugs to money. But I kept hoping he'd change." Encounters like these breed a cycle of fighting and sex, terror and turn-off—and they are often fueled by alcohol or drugs, which add another layer of horror and lack of control.

Women also speak of emotional and physical neglect, which has its own continuum and its own stranglehold on desire. Neglect that begins in child-hood can trigger a lifelong desperation for all that was missed out on: love, touch, affection, food, clothing, education, comfort. If this is your story, you may find yourself unclear about what might nourish you now—in all ways, including sexual. Neglect in our adult relationships can also affect desire. I'm remembering a client whose photographer husband constantly took pictures of everyone except her. Once she understood that this was only one of the ways he was intentionally overlooking her, she was able to frame it as a form of abuse—by systematic omission.

"It's All My Fault"

Despite the well-publicized effects of trauma and abuse, it often comes as a surprise to women that their past experiences have any bearing on their present problems with sexual desire. So many survivors blame themselves for their lack of sexual interest and feeling. I cannot count the number of clients who come into my sex therapy office asking: "Doctor, what's wrong with *me*?" A nurse nearing retirement age relates that she'd suffered repeated sexual violence, beginning with her father, yet she still faults herself for her lack of desire, complaining that she can't stay in the sexual moment long enough to fully absorb good feelings: "I've had orgasms and I've felt intense pleasure, but I'm never totally unaware. Nor totally con-nected. Part of me hangs back from everything and everyone."

The New York editor quoted earlier says she also struggles with fall-out from the traumas of her past. Yet she never points a finger at her tor-mentors—she points only at herself. She sees herself as "your average Jewish neurotic baby-boomer artist," with a long string of dysfunctional behaviors:

This hole in my heart is the same hole I try to fill with sex or romance. Perhaps I just use sex in an attempt to heal old wounds. After I've been with someone a few months I regress to a childlike demeanor, although I date much younger men. Other warning signs are that I keep relationships at bay with almost pathological jealousy, and I've never felt truly committed to anyone.

Responses to abuse and violence may have other complexities. Some women discover that their memories can be a source not only of disgust and avoidance but also of sexual excitement. But this is an admission few women make because they feel ashamed, and scared that feeling this way marks them as perverts—reflecting again the notion that it's the victims who are at fault. Here's how one woman puts it.

My first sexual experience occurred at the age of three. A thirteen-year-old boy sexually molested me in a car parked in our back alley. The two things I remember feeling about that experience are: (1) I liked it. (2) It was wrong.

But confusing as it seems, even unwanted sexual attention may make us feel special, and even unwanted stimulation may be physically arousing. For some survivors, arousal can become so intertwined with violence that they actually desire what hurts and humiliates. They describe seeking sexual encounters that result in black eyes, bruised kidneys, trampled self-esteem, rape.

Other survivors manage to incorporate the "excitement" of those abusive experiences in ways that are much less destructive, even pleasure-enhancing. They reframe their memories of abuse into their sexual fantasies—as scenes of intrigue and danger. They transpose them into inventive sex play such as spanking, bondage, and dominance-submission games. Many sex therapists feel both fantasy and S/M behaviors can be innovative outlets for sexual desire, especially when entered into with awareness. To read a myth-breaking collection about S/M behaviors, scripts, and code words that goes where most sex researchers fear to tread, see *Sadomasochism: Powerful Pleasures* by Peggy Kleinplatz and Charles Moser.

Pleasure Anxiety
The Fear of Feeling Good

Too many of us live out our lives afraid of feeling good. We're afraid to ask for what we want, and we're afraid to enjoy it—even when pleasure knocks at our door with a bouquet of roses and begs to come in. We get adept at keeping pleasure at bay with a barrage of head noises: "I'll feel exposed." "I'll be too vulnerable." "I'll lose control." "I don't want them to think I'm a loose woman." "I'll never be able to please a partner." "I don't deserve it." For some women there's no stopping this internal static—and this is especially true for those of us with backgrounds of abuse.

More than half a century ago, psychoanalyst Wilhelm Reich, a colleague of Freud and the founder of bioenergetic therapy, recognized that many of his patients shared a fear of feeling good. He labeled it "pleasure anxiety." What he had discovered by careful questioning was that the desire for sexual pleasure and ecstasy was sometimes more terrifying than the threat of rejection, pain, or even death. He observed this terror in adults who'd grown up in families that were physically and emotionally abusive—many of them hid their actions behind masks of self-righteous discipline. He also observed this degree of terror in adults whose families had routinely withheld affection (just the kind of don't-touch family I grew up in, I thought, when I first discovered Reich). He called these families "factories of repression," and saw them as training grounds for sexual dysfunction, disconnection, joylessness, and violence, especially toward women.

Reich also famously observed the cultural implications of pleasure anxiety. He saw that the inability to embrace sexual pleasure sprang directly from a dominator society that is driven by control and violence—conditions that abounded in fascist Germany where he lived in the 1930s. Reich's notion that pleasure anxiety is embedded in the culture means that it can act systemically and epidemically. And here, it's important for women with happy childhood memories to listen up—your sexual response may be inhibited even when your personal upbringing seems to have been sex-positive and appropriate.

It's plain to see how pleasure anxiety might be a pervasive problem, particularly for women raised in dominator families. But it doesn't take sexual abuse or an openly fascist state to create this kind of personal dysfunction. We may absorb the fear of feeling good directly from the times we live in. Overwork, stress, financial worries, inadequate sex education—these might not be classified as abuse, but they can all sap our sexual desire. We could add war to this list as well, if we're willing to recognize that damage to our individual lives is not only a result of a dominator culture, but also serves to perpetuate a broader social trauma.

To add to the confusion, today's society is highly sexualized. Everywhere you look, there's some kind of feel-good goal—more money, more speed, more sugar. The sexual goals are all about intercourse, not about the kind of pleasure that nourishes our spirits as well as our bodies. Couple this goal of sensation with the widespread notion that women are supposed to be less sexual than men, and it's no wonder so many of us say "Ouch!"

How We Suppress Sexual Desire
Armor, Denial, Dissociation, Faking It

It's natural to develop defenses against abuse and other assaults on our sexual sensibilities. Over my years as a sex therapist, I've learned how infinitely resourceful women can be in keeping sexual desire at bay. Some of us develop the fine art of sexual gatekeeping so we can stop the flow of feeling before it overwhelms us, or even touches us. We stuff ourselves with food. We use alcohol to mimic warmth and comfort. We use sugar and caffeine to mimic heart-racing excitement. We watch sitcoms to mimic human relationship and reality shows to mimic our basic instincts for survival. We spend hours at the gym, plodding out our frustrations on the treadmill. We shop. An inveterate shopper describes how she substitutes "retail therapy" for the emptiness that occurs when she can't feel good feelings about sex:

> I think most of us probably spend tons of energy shutting out pleasure—feelings of connectedness to our world and others.

Then spend lots of money trying to get well, feel better, make sense of our lives.

ARMOR
"YOU CAN'T FIND ME."

Some women develop an effective suit of armor against all good feelings. The armor can feel quite literal. Maybe you pack on weight and disappear under layers of fat. Maybe you develop joint problems and can't move fluidly. The armor can be invisible, too. Emotional armor keeps you from opening your heart. Mental armor keeps your thoughts and fantasies on the straight and narrow. Spiritual armor separates you from your deepest longings. All this self-imposed armor keeps others out—but it traps you inside as well. You may have worn it so long that it functions like a second skin—or heart, or soul.

Your personal armor protects you from much more than pain. It also protects you from fully feeling pleasure. It helps you maintain the kind of self-control that makes you a fabulous emergency-room nurse or war hero. But armoring yourself against feeling good doesn't serve you well if you're trying to relate intimately with a partner and bring desire back into your life. And if your partner has on a full suit of armor, too, it can be impossible to make real contact. Think about it. You're like a couple of armadillos trying to make a go of it in bed.

DENIAL
"DON'T TALK, DON'T TOUCH, DON'T FEEL."

Another primary form of defense against sexual desire is denial of its existence. As long as you can keep yourself from talking, touching, or feeling, you can bypass the desire for just about anything, including sexual pleasure. Here's how a physician's assistant says denial allowed her to survive her marital past—as she deliberately shelved her sexual feelings well into her sixties.

> I had a bad marriage. I do have desire but never had anyone to fulfill me. There are many people in this world who never have sex and are happy and content. I'm sure it must be nice, but sex is not a must for a nice life.

Shifting her focus away from sexual pleasure may have separated this woman from a history she'd rather forget. This technique may work well for her, but it's not for everyone. Clearly it didn't help her move along the path to rich and vibrant partnership, which is what so many women tell me they want. Her story is an example of how it's possible to swallow societal messages whole and end up believing that a "nice" life of marginal love and libid is all we can ever hope for.

The truth is, denial can wreak havoc with sexual desire no matter what kind of relationship you choose. A social worker displays the other side of sexual denial—seeking "mega-sensation" but turning a blind eye to the consequences. She says she found herself craving extraordinary sexual risks just so she could feel something. She chose dangerous settings, dangerous partners, unprotected sex with potentially abusive and emotionally unavailable men and women.

> The most fulfilling sexual experiences of my life were several ménage à trois situations I was involved in with two men, going to swingers clubs where I could fulfill my danger fantasies and engage in sex with women, but not feel like I was cheating on my partner.

The quality of her sexual play is different from the polyamorous lifestyles outlined in chapter 9—where all the partners agree to communicate about the sexual interactions and ensure that they're safe and aboveboard. While there are poly partners who engage in ménages à trois (and possibly ménages à *more*), the motivation in those relationships is not to court risk and danger, but to develop ways of being in the world that open and expand sexual desire.

What I've found crucial for women to understand about denial is that sexual desire is connected to our whole lives. We have infinite choices about where—and how—we choose to focus our energy. The more conscious we can be of our feelings, the more likely we are to make choices that keep us vital—both in and out of the bedroom.

DISSOCIATION
"DISAPPEARING, TAKING A POWDER, GOING POOF"

When feeling good triggers flashbacks of extreme pain and humiliation, some women remove themselves from the scene by dissociating—that is, they split off mentally from their experience, body, mind, heart, and spirit. Remember the woman in chapter 3 who makes shopping lists in her head during sex? This is a gentle example of splitting. Other women have told me they watch TV while their husbands "do their business," or fantasize about a totally different partner, or take themselves into another realm entirely. For instance, a survivor client constructed a warren of places in her mind where she hid from sexual feelings. It took years of therapy and an incredibly supportive mate before she could connect with genuine feelings of sexual desire. Dissociating in certain situations isn't necessarily a bad thing. Clearly, moving away from what hurts is a healthy instinct. But blocking out pain completely and on a regular basis cuts down on your ability to feel anything, including joy.

Some women with histories of sexual abuse remain permanently dissociated—diagnosed with what used to be called multiple personality and is now called dissociative identity disorder (DID). By either name, it means that you fragment yourself into a number of separate identities to help you escape from trauma, or cope with it. Health writer Jane Hyman conducted in-depth interviews with eleven of these women, all successful professionals. Her book *I Am More Than One* tells the story of how they function in various aspects of their lives. I especially remember the story of "Barbara," a social worker whose way of enduring the terrors from her gruesome childhood was to develop a cadre of personalities who continue to help her handle difficult situations in the present. When the adult Barbara begins to feel overwhelmed with sexual sensations, she relies on Slut Girl, the personality whose function is to have fun. Slut Girl loves sex and will happily have it with anyone who asks. The system works because Barbara's other personalities keep Slut Girl from making unwise choices and getting into trouble.

Not all of us can call on an internal cast of characters to monitor our sexual interactions. But Barbara's story is a graphic reminder that desire is complex and may involve more than one approach, more than one set of skills or belief systems. Her study also underscores that bringing sexual desire back from limbo may mean creating safe boundaries as well as opening up to pleasure. The ability to call on multiple facets of the personality is honored in indigenous cultures as a spiritual gift. Although our culture pathologizes this way of dealing with unendurable pain, for some women it can lead to innovative ways to connect with the complex paths to sexual desire.

FAKING DESIRE AND INTIMACY

We've all heard about faking orgasm. Forty-eight percent of American women do it, says a 2004 ABC News poll; 72 percent, says the online magazine *Slate* in its 2000 orgasm survey. Sex therapist Carol Ellison reports about 70 percent in her book *Women's Sexualities,* which is based on survey responses she gathered from over two thousand women. Some of these women said they'd faked it once, writes Ellison, and some "countless" or "a bazillion" times. One woman drew an infinity sign as her answer. Their reasons for faking? Mostly to get sex over with more quickly, or to stroke their partners' egos.

But what about faking sexual desire? Or faking sexual closeness and intimacy? This is what I hear from numerous women who come to me for therapy. This level of faking can creep toxically into all aspects of our relationships to undermine openhearted honesty and sharing—which are primary qualities that make sex (and everything else) meaningful. However unconscious or even well-meaning, it may be that any degree of faking represents a selling out of right relationship with our partners and also ourselves.

Why do women fake it? Like Ellison's respondents, we fake it to please our partners and get it over with. As Reich observed, we fake it because we're afraid to feel the full range of pleasure. Some of us fake it in an attempt to spice up Johnny-one-note sex that never goes beyond intercourse. Some of us fake it because we can't access our own feelings so we mimic the sex-kitten images we see on late-night TV. Some of us fake it because we don't feel the same lust that pulsed through every pore when we first fell madly in love—and we want to make ourselves believe we're still that youthful and lusty. Some of us fake it in an earnest effort to feel more, to quicken those pulses, to make things good again—to "fake it till we make it," as the saying goes. And some of us fake it because we're so needy for emotional connection that we can't see beyond our fear that we'll never get what we want. One client confided, "I've faked my way through my whole life because I was scared if I told the truth they'd just laugh at me, then I'd die of shame."

Faking can get us over some rough spots—but over the long term it undermines our capacity for spontaneity and innovation. When we keep repeating the same script, we miss what's happening in the present. There's a Stepford-wife quality to faking desire and intimacy—as if our capacity for pleasure has been replaced by a computer chip that cries out "Oh God!" at specified intervals. Our internal data banks may briefly flare, but we don't feel moved or satisfied or authentic.

Healing after Trauma
Recognizing Our True Allies

Despite the grim truths about sexual abuse and the toll it can take on sexual desire, there is hope. Countless women have been able to find remarkable and courageous ways to create enough light to dissolve their personal shadows. Some seek recovery through therapy—to help them move through their fear and rage and connect with joy. Some seek recovery through spiritual study and practice. Many survivors are drawn to Eastern philosophies and religions. Buddhism, especially, opens up the idea that suffering is an unavoidable aspect of the human condition—and that it can be mitigated through cultivating awareness and compassion for ourselves and others.

For other women, twelve-step recovery programs have proven crucial to their healing path. An accountant confides that her recovery from drinking and smoking pot allowed her to uncover feelings and sensations she'd buried until she was in her forties. "It allowed me to like myself." Coincidentally, she also fell in love with a man who believed sex was about connection and not just about "thrusting and coming."

"THE LOVE OF A GOOD PARTNER . . ."

A powerful source of recovery and healing comes directly from the partnerships women develop. One woman who responded to my ISIS survey affirms that it was "intense spiritual connectedness" with her present partner that helped her heal from child sexual abuse and from gang rape as an adult. This partnership provided her with "unconditional positive regard and love." An art gallery administrator concurs. She says the buoyancy she experiences in her present relationship helped her make a conscious decision to move beyond negativity she'd carried with her since early girlhood. It took years of experimenting with her "dark side" and feeding her depression with "quasi and completely destructive sex" before she understood that one-night stands were a setup for disaster—because what she longed for was intimacy, not just sensation.

> I "bottomed out" with a borderline individual—recovering drug addict, etc., etc. And I realized it was time to reformat my psyche and libido and let my poor little heart overcome its terror of love.

For some women, finding the love of a good partner may take more than one try. A Seattle homemaker illustrates how important it is to persevere; that it's possible to overcome sex negativity and abuse that have skewed our sexual attitudes long before we're adults:

> When I was young, I lived in a house where no one kissed, hugged, or touched. I never knew about sex, as it was "taboo." On my wedding day, my mother told me "It takes about ten or fifteen minutes. Just lie there and take whatever he does. After that you can take a shower." My uncle molested me when I was thirteen. My mother caught him in the act and banned him from the house. I was not allowed to talk about the experience.

She goes on—to illustrate the stunning optimism that can shine through a life of hardship.

> My first husband taught me the pleasures of sex, and the first years of our marriage were beautiful. After he became addicted to drugs, however, he became abusive and our sexual life was a nightmare. Once he "sold" my "services" for a bag of H [heroin]. I was repeatedly sodomized and needed surgical repair. My second husband unfortunately became impotent for the last three years of our marriage before he died.

My third husband has been "heaven-sent." It has been with him that I've discovered that spirituality and sex need not be separated and that the core of each of us is the essence of the universe—love. When we come together physically, it's as if the Goddess and the God are there also. Although we've only been together six years, we've never had an argument. Each time we make love it is total ecstasy spiritually, mentally, and physically. For the first time in my life I understand the concept: "The two become one flesh." We also become one with the Great All, *Love.*

Physical love is the deepest expression of the creator we can experience on this plane of existence.

In this woman's story there is a crucial message for all of us who long for a relationship that nourishes and satisfies: Don't give up and give in to the notion that your life is over because you were forced to endure an unendurable past. Her story gives us a glimpse into another legacy of abuse and trauma—the immense gratitude for love and healthy sexual relationship when they finally enter our lives.

"WHEN OUR HEARTS BREAK, LIGHT SHINES IN . . ."

Some women say that they've actually been able to use their negative experiences as a path to the joy of the sexual desire they seek. A West Coast psychologist reports that her recovery process opened her to explore the connections between sex and spirit:

> While in treatment for "adults molested as children" I realized the "gift" of being molested . . . once I cleared the anger, shame, hatred. It forced me to love my body and soul for its life force, pleasure, creativity, and power.

When our hearts break, says a Sufi teaching, this allows more light to shine in, and ultimately more love to shine in, too. Spiritual healers the world over teach us that hurt, pain, craziness, and dismemberment are often spiritual initiations—that is, they crack the shell of our egos to expose the deepest truths and surest routes to healing. Even the ancient goddesses weren't immune. Inanna, the Sumerian goddess of sex and fertility, had to embark on a grisly underworld journey to reclaim her identity, her sacred marriage, and her royal trappings as the "hot-limbed" Great Mother.

A colleague recently wrote to tell me how the last few years have led her into her own underworld journey. Heartbreak, betrayal, and even violation have helped to expand her—instead of constrict or fragment her. She now has the sense that she's newly reborn from a cosmic birth canal.

> When I've gone into the depths of my heart, I emerge with a much bigger capacity to love—including more compassion for my self and the other, more freedom to love and be loved again, and more—words don't match the experience. It's a change in consciousness about self and other, and hence a full circle—to LIGHT.

For some women, recovering sexual desire after abuse or trauma requires understanding the context of both their negative and their positive experiences—to regain "balance and growth, joy and pleasure," says another woman. She speaks of "the things which guide us when times are dark, make life worth living when it's not—and make me extremely dangerous to men and machines when I'm horny."

The story of a teacher who attended one of my ISIS workshops demonstrates how helpful it can sometimes be to understand our negative experiences in the most concrete way possible. She'd come to the workshop to explore the many sexual traumas of her childhood—and she'd brought with her a fist-sized black rock to represent the heaviness of these traumas. All the abuse had occurred in the family cabin at the edge of a lake, a place she hadn't revisited for almost thirty years. After the workshop, she took her rock with her and returned to that cabin. She stood outside and looked through the bedroom window to where the sexual abuse had happened. She allowed herself to relive the seduction, the fear, the helplessness, "all the energy of all those memories."

She expected to feel agony and confusion—after all, she'd continued to live with them every day for decades. But peering into that window she felt something else, too—and it astonished her. She was flooded with memories of warmth and nurturing. She breathed deeply and allowed herself to remember how she'd sometimes enjoyed those special attentions in the dark—the fondling, and the orgasms, which she suddenly realized had excited her fully as much as they shamed her.

It wasn't until she'd run through her full spectrum of feelings that she finally comprehended the mind-numbing rage she'd been holding on to all these years—about being overpowered, forced, trapped, even trapped into enjoying her orgasms. She let herself yell and rant about the "boundary-hopping invasions" that had robbed her of her childhood. She looked at the black rock in her hand and knew what she needed to do to loosen the grip of those memories so she could move on.

Here is part of a letter she sent to our group after her experience:

> I got really clear that the rock belongs in the bottom of the lake. I bound all of that negativity into the rock, and intended for each and every person who violated me to take back their own energy, and I walked to the shore of the lake and hurled that blessed rock out into the middle of the lake in a surefire act of release, and letting go.

Hurling her rock of negativity into the family lake was a symbolic act to be sure. But for her it was also a concrete act of trust and hope. And it was transformative. It was an act that released from her body and spirit what she says years of psychotherapy had never been able to dislodge. "Negative long-standing energy blocks and memories have been removed and I indeed feel like a whole new person."

Exploring Your Sexual Desire
Using the ISIS Wheel to Begin Healing from Trauma

How do you take your sexual desire back from the grip of all the defenses you may have developed over the years? You begin by allowing yourself to feel, to expand, to reach out beyond how you were defined in the past. Some women do all this in a rush—and some need to start slowly. I usually suggest beginning on the mental path of the ISIS Wheel—because this is where it's possible for you to exercise a good deal of cognitive control and support, which is especially important after a history of trauma.

THE MENTAL PATH TO RECLAIMING SEXUAL DESIRE
WAKING UP YOUR MIND

Begin by asking yourself these questions: When is it safe to let down my guard, take off my armor against feeling sexual desire—When I fall in love? When my kids grow up? When I'm old enough to collect social security? The timing is different for everyone. Let yourself be clear about what's right for you. Maybe the timing is never. If that's your choice, honor it—as long as it truly is a choice and not something you're doing only to please someone else.

Suppose you decide that the time to reclaim sexual desire is now—how do you begin to think about this? One method I've used successfully comes from Fritz Perls, the Gestalt guru who spent his last years helping a generation of seekers move beyond their stuck places, or "impasses," as he called them. He created a brilliant and simple equation to help us conceptualize how to expand beyond our sticking points. It goes like this:

$$\frac{\text{Awareness} + \text{Risk-taking}}{\text{Growth}}$$

"Awareness plus risk-taking equals growth." Those five words are easy to say—but much harder to put into daily practice. Think about it. Until you have awareness of both your abuse *and* your sexual desire, taking risks can be foolhardy—potentially unsafe to yourself and others, as it was for the woman quoted earlier who engaged in unsafe sex to fulfill her danger fantasies.

Sometimes the first inkling of awareness is when you open a little chink in the armor you've constructed around yourself and peek through to the outside. From your vantage point on the mental path of the ISIS Wheel make a list of what might make it safe for you to open up this chink an inch or two more and take some carefully calculated risks.

Some items women have written on their lists include:

"I am more powerful as an adult than I was when I was a child."

"I know my partner cares deeply about me."

"I know I can always jump back into my armor if I get too scared."

You can discuss your list with your partner and with others. You can also read some of the wonderful books on how to recognize abuse and heal its effects. Wendy Maltz is one of the sex therapists who writes wisely and compassionately about the subject. Her book *The Sexual Healing Journey* is a classic on how to reclaim positive sexual feelings after a history of abuse. Other books I regularly recommend are *The Courage to Heal* by Ellen Bass and Laura Davis and *Trauma and Recovery* by Judith Herman.

But awareness means more than intellectual acknowledgment. Information about sexual desire needs to radiate beyond your capacity for logic and reason. The next step in awareness is to bring this knowledge into your emotional feelings, into your heart.

THE EMOTIONAL PATH TO RECLAIMING SEXUAL DESIRE
WAKING UP YOUR FEELINGS

For most of us, tapping into our emotions is the riskiest part of reclaiming sexual desire—especially risky after a history of sexual abuse. My shamanic teacher, Oscar Miro-Quesada, states that the longest journey in the world is the journey from the head to the heart. Yet he also asserts that we'll probably stay only partly alive if we never risk taking that journey.

So we need emotional risk-taking along with intellectual awareness. One simple exercise comes from my Gestalt therapy training—Perls again. Try it. This is your opportunity to take full responsibility for your loss of desire—and also to take responsibility for doing all you can to reclaim it.

It's a simple sentence completion. You can do this exercise by yourself—and you may double the impact if you do it with a partner. You get more ideas. You also get to give and receive feedback. The important thing is to *feel* what you're saying.

Here's sentence number one:

"I can turn off my sexual desire by . . ."

Complete this sentence over and over until you run out of creative ideas. You can journal, you can draw pictures, you can meditate—whatever helps you complete this sentence by indicating all the ways that are true for you.

Here are some ways women have completed this sentence:

> "I can turn off my sexual desire by telling myself that my body is ugly."

> "I can turn off my sexual desire by obsessing about awful events from the past."

> "I can turn off my sexual desire by imagining that something terrible will happen to me if I let go of control."

> "I can turn off my sexual desire by talking instead of feeling."

Here's the second sentence for you to complete:

"I can turn *on* my sexual desire by . . ."

This is your opportunity to take responsibility for the active steps you can take to change your situation in a positive way. Say all the things that are true for you. You may surprise yourself with the number of options you come up with.

Here are some ways women have completed the sentence:

> "I can turn on my sexual desire by having a massage."

> "I can turn on my sexual desire by looking into my partner's eyes."

> "I can turn on my sexual desire by remembering the last time I felt really good."

> "I can turn on my sexual desire by forgiving myself for being scared."

Again, review your list with yourself (and your partner)—and consider which of these ideas you'd be willing to put into practice. And let yourself feel your feelings.

THE PHYSICAL PATH TO RECLAIMING SEXUAL DESIRE
WAKING UP YOUR BODY

One easy way to wake up your body is to brush every inch you can reach with a bath brush before you take a shower—and also during your shower. This gets your blood flowing to the surface of your skin, which helps you feel more alive. Also, your brush strokes join each part of you to each other part of you—so that your body remembers what it feels like to be connected from head to toe, from hand to heart, from belly to genitals.

You can intensify this wake-up call by rubbing yourself all over with a mixture of sea salt and baking soda (half-and-half). Then rinse off until you're squeaky clean. Now slather on the most delicious oil or lotion you have and luxuriate in your silky skin.

This wake-up-your-body routine can feel even better with a partner—even if it's not your intimate partner. My favorite way to enjoy the salt rub is outdoors in the summer where the warm breezes can caress my skin—preferably in a shower by the ocean on a sunny day. Mmmmmmm.

Healing with your own hands. When your body feels clean and alive is a wonderful time to wake it up even more by using an age-old method of healing touch—I learned this from Maril and Jim Crabtree, who teach it at Core Star, their Kansas City center for healing. But you don't need to possess any special skills to benefit from it—just warm hands and an intention for feeling good.

Start by sitting or lying in a comfortable spot, and close your eyes. Place your hands on a part of your body that you believe carries the wounds of your abuse. Perhaps it's your heart, or your belly. Perhaps it's your vagina or your breasts. There may be more than one spot, and it's important that you eventually reach every one of them—but for now, let's start with just one. Touch that place now—even if it's a place where outward wounds didn't show.

Wherever it is, lay your hands on that wounded place now—just as you might reach out to comfort a baby who's crying herself to sleep.

Let yourself feel the tears flow into your hands—and imagine you can pull all the hurt out with your fingers.

Then shake out your hands until they're free of hurt and tears and place them back on your body. Now let yourself feel the vulnerability and sweetness that's underneath the wounding.

Remember (or imagine) how this wounded place felt when it was whole and vibrant—before it sustained the hurt. See yourself as a playful innocent child—or whatever positive image is true for you.

Now imagine that you can weave that positive image back into your wounded place, as if you're repairing a fabric that has been torn.

Take your time doing this—and spend some time in open attention afterward. Notice what you feel in your body when you lay healing hands on yourself.

THE SPIRITUAL PATH TO RECLAIMING SEXUAL DESIRE
EXORCISING YOUR FEAR AND WAKING UP YOUR SELF

For many women, especially abuse survivors, shedding fear may be a crucial part of the prescription for the return of sexual desire—so that we can expand our sense of self, of love, of creativity, altruism, and hope.

Exorcising fear in a concrete way is part of a time-honored healing tradition of allying with divine energy. Alberto Villoldo is a shamanic "earthkeeper" who writes movingly about this tradition in *The Four Insights*. He tells of a ritual he uses to help his students move beyond fear of feeling, and fear of death. He teaches them how to transfer their fears into a symbolic stone and then has them cast that stone into the sacred Jaguar Lagoon high in the Peruvian Andes.

We've already seen the power of a similar ritual in the story of the teacher who cast her abuses into the family lake. This was a spontaneous act on her part. But you can use the intent behind her story to create a powerful experience for yourself.

Find a stone to represent the negative experiences that are holding back your joy of sexual pleasure. Hold this stone to your lips and blow into it your feelings about all the times sexual desire has died for you—take as much time as you need. And also blow into it your fears of opening to all the pleasure you deserve in your life now. This stone now holds the energy of all those negative memories.

Don't get rid of this stone just yet. Keep it with you and carry it everywhere you go—for as long as you feel you need to hold on to all that negativity in your life. Notice how you feel carrying it with you. Is it awkward? Is it a responsibility? Is it heavy? How do you explain to your partner that you have to keep this stone between you in bed?

When you're ready to let go of the negativities, prepare yourself to release your stone. Carry it with you to a body of water that you believe has the ability to transform. Then with all your intention for healing, cast your stone into the water.

I'm not suggesting that simply throwing a stone is going to magically erase the traumas of your past and bring back light, hope, and sexual desire. But I am reminding you that desire is complex—and that by using the stone (or some of the other rituals we've talked about to exorcise fear) you can connect focused spiritual intention with focused attention to your body, heart, and mind. You may be surprised and delighted by the kinds of desire that begin to return to your life.

Part Three

∞

EXPANDING *Your* BELIEFS
about SEXUAL DESIRE

What does it feel like to connect sexuality and spirituality?

I feel like there's a great void in my chest and heart—all negative emotions are being cleared and pulled out into the atmosphere while a deep concrete sense of belonging and love begins to take its place and permeate outward into the other's soul. You forget any imperfections you may have and have faith in the love and person you are with. There is joy and peace as well as excitement and lust. Sometimes it's so good you could cry.

—*Twenty-three-year-old waitress from Olympia, Washington*

Feeling humble and vulnerable in the face of the awesome miracles of life and love. To love and be loved—by another human being or God—is a profound gift. To remain small and reverential in the face of it all keeps me connected to bliss.

—*Thirty-seven-year-old businesswoman from Cummington, Massachusetts*

I have, in the last two years, discovered sexuality to be a doorway to amazing cosmic experiences—experiences of oneness, not with my partner so much as with the universe—becoming light, a starry night, an ocean of love, pleasure itself. I feel altered—grounded, very peaceful and relaxed for days afterward.

—*Forty-seven-year-old midwife from Boise, Idaho*

When I have a strong orgasm, my body dissolves into light and I sense an opening in the third eye area—an opening into unconditional love and a feeling of oneness with all. All fears and worries are forgotten. In fact, it seems that when I am having frequent and full lovemaking I rarely experience stress and overwhelming worries and fears. It has the strength of prayer—it is a body prayer to love.

—*Fifty-year-old therapist from Bozeman, Montana*

12

SACRED UNION
The Desire for Connection and Meaning

WOMEN'S STORIES REVEAL just how complex sexual desire can be. Its return involves a multifaceted journey, not just a trip to your drugstore to pick up a prescription for hormones or antidepressants. It means acknowledging your emotions and your thoughts as well as your physical sensations. It means honoring your memories and dreams as well as your here-and-now experiences. It means seeking clarity in your relationships—not only with your partner, but with yourself. Sometimes it means reaching deep into your own center and beyond—as if sexual desire is a launching pad for sacred connection and meaning.

What does "sacred" mean in the context of your sexual desire? This is a tough question for some of us because we've been so conditioned to think of sexuality and spirituality as separate. Yet there are women who assert that sex is a path to the divine. They say connecting sex and spirit feels like waking up to the cosmos—sometimes all at once, sometimes bit by bit.

For some women the idea of sacred sex has to do with worship and prayer—acknowledging that there's an intensely loving higher power that guides every aspect of their relationships, including sexual desire. Other women describe sacred sex as a feeling of oneness with their partners, the urge to connect through the heart, not just the genitals. Still other women see spiritual connection in qualities like honesty, love, altruism, and vitality that are woven into the everyday fabric of their relationships. Women who talk about sacred sex speak of letting go of old patterns that keep them disconnected from themselves and their partners. They speak of taking on a balance and grace that informs the daily workings of their lives.

All these descriptions invest desire with feeling and vibrations that are beyond purely physical sensation. This kind of experience is what so many of my women clients say they find missing in their own sexual relationships—and what they say so many of their male partners just don't seem to get: "He tells me he thinks everything's fine the way it is." What these women long for is for sexual connection that moves them to reach beyond themselves for deep and lasting meaning.

The truth is, all of our sexual relationships have meaning. Some are more meaningful than others. Falling madly in love can change the trajectory of your whole life. A lifelong partnership affects every aspect of your existence. But even when sexual encounters seem to be casual or fleeting, they may have much to teach about our own responses. Some teach about love, commitment, and pleasure. Others teach about loneliness, disconnection, and pain.

The surface lessons are usually pretty clear. But if you dig deep enough, any of our sexual relationships may include a spiritual dimension that's beyond our cognitive understanding. Many women say they have no adequate words to explain this dimension, they just know it's there.

It's no wonder words fail us. This spiritual dimension of sexual relationship is a confluence of energies, not of thoughts or sensations. You can't explain it in a logical way. It doesn't depend on how many times you "do it" or how many orgasms you achieve. You can't increase it by using testosterone patches, vaginal dilators, or a Kegelmaster that strengthens the muscles of your pelvic floor. You can't touch it, count it, or measure it. It belongs in the realm of "irrational facts," to requote Carl Jung's wonderful phrase about spiritual experience. Though neuroscientists are homing in on explanations that include a clearer understanding of how hormones and neuropeptides affect our sexual desire, love, and well-being, the spiritual nature of sexual desire is still difficult to describe.

Yet our spirituality speaks to us in a universally understood language—in our overall zest for life as well as for sexual pleasure, in our capacity for joy. It's central to whatever draws us to one another heart to heart. It's part of what enables us to light up in each other's presence. When desire is flowing, this spiritual dimension is likely to be part of the flow. When desire is flagging, connecting with spirit may help you revive it.

When Sexual Union Is Sacred

The phrase "sacred union" is routinely used to describe the religious sacrament of marriage. But it's much more. Sacred union can appear in a lavish smorgasbord of relationships, with or without religious validation. Women talk about experiencing a sense of sacred union in their straight marriages, gay marriages, and marriages of convenience. They talk about sacred union in monogamous commitment and serial monogamy, in intimate friendships and spiritual partnerships. They talk about it in dating, affairs, casual encounters, and polyamory. And they talk about it in the relationships they have with themselves—a relationship that's fundamental to any we form with an intimate other—as we've seen illustrated in chapter 5.

About nine in every ten respondents of my ISIS survey use the term "oneness" to describe their feelings about sacred union. Some women— and men—see sacred union as a mystical meeting of body, mind, heart, and soul. Some say it's a soul connection with their partners. And some say it's a connection with themselves, their partners, and also something beyond, whether they name that something nature, God, Goddess, Higher Power, Spirit, or Universal Energy.

Some women say sexual energy can create a kind of relationship in and of itself. A thirty-two-year-old artist and stay-at-home mom from North Carolina deliciously reports such a relationship. On good days, she says, a sense of sex and spirit seems to pervade every aspect of her life—as if sexual desire connects her with the rhythms of nature and spirit and all that is.

> Some of my best "sex" has been creating beauty in the world in art, writing, and gardening—sharing gifts from Spirit. Sacred sex is spiritual and not just found in intercourse. It's all around, in everything we see, hear, smell, touch, taste. Honey is sex. A fresh warm strawberry is sex. Living is a sacred sexual experience.

In my workshops, I often ask women to read this passage aloud. Hearing a real live voice proclaim the "honey" of sexual desire, the freshness and warmth and immanence of our sensual sexual selves, invariably moves other women to open up with their own stories of connection and meaning. And when we talk together about the intricate layers of our sexual desires, it gives us support to imagine that our own experiences make a difference. I encourage this kind of free-flowing conversation that ensues about sex and spirit. I believe our stories are central to our creating a new conversation about sexual desire—one that transcends performance and scoring.

How Spirituality Meets Desire
Creating a Launching Pad for Meaningful Sex

If sexual desire means attraction to one another and spirituality means reaching beyond ourselves, how do these two concepts meet? And what does the meeting entail?

Spirituality meets desire in love, which is a universal component of sacred union—nearly nine of every ten women who responded to my ISIS survey say love is essential for sexual satisfaction. The kind of love that promotes sacred sexual union involves opening your heart—both to give and receive. It involves empathy, the ability to feel what your partner is feeling. It also involves compassion, the ability to affirm each other even in the face of guilt, shame, depression, and anxiety about "doing it right."

Spirituality meets desire in the quality of attention we focus on one another. Women say they feel that attention through touch, listening, and eye contact. "Just by him looking at me with such passion and love, I feel like he's inside me even when he's not," says a newly married accountant. And they feel that attention through listening to their own internal openings, their own rhythms. Focused attention can feel like reverence. The return of desire can feel like worship. It can feel like sacred presence—totally absorbed in the moment, yet timeless, even eternal.

Spirituality meets desire in the intensity of our passion. It's evident in the vitality we exude when we're around each other, in our ability to feel enthusiasm and even awe. A twenty-one-year-old speaks of the first time she experienced passionate sex.

> A fire was lit within my soul. I was doing an ancient dance of life. I felt something deep within myself awaken. I felt raw and

natural. I became the animal, pure, real, and free. The next day I felt transformed. I knew I had truly become a woman.

Spirituality meets desire in safety. I'm not talking about boring predictability. I'm talking about creating a haven for each other so that you can let down your guard without fear of hurt or dismissal. As one ISIS respondent remarks, "He reveled in my sexuality, there was never a hint or whisper of shame." This bespeaks commitment—not necessarily the till-death-do-us-part kind of commitment, though some women do want and need this. Rather, it's a commitment to knowing all there is about yourself and each other—and being open to surprise.

Spirituality meets desire in trusting relationships. Sexual honesty means being clear about commitments—is this a monogamous relationship? Is it open, or polyamorous? If so, what are your agreements around other sexual partners? Sexual honesty means asking for what you want, not making your partner guess and then pulling back because it wasn't right. It means being open with yourself as well as your partner—allowing yourself to become vulnerable enough to melt into the truth, even when it might feel easier to skirt around the truth or tell a lie.

Spirituality meets desire in kissing. Ah, kissing. Many women say mouth-to-mouth feels like heart-to-heart—and far more intimate than intercourse. This isn't just the stuff of romance novels and grainy old movies. Eight in ten ISIS women say kissing soulfully is what helps make sex spiritual for them. "Moving, profound, and soul-shattering" is how one woman describes her lover's kisses.

Spirituality meets desire in our ability to share our feelings—and share them deeply. Our heart's yearnings. Our most embarrassing moments. Our profound needs. Our dark secrets. Our erotic fantasies. Our inner visions—which may be just as scary to share as our secrets and fantasies. The list is endless. We can even engage in deep sharing long-distance. One woman says she got to know her mate when he was stationed in Europe—they poured out their souls in letters to each other, exposing every detail of each other's lives. Many women speak of reaching each other's core through gift-giving, parenting their kids, tenderness, and humor. Seven in ten ISIS women say it's laughing together that helps spark sexual desire.

Spirituality meets desire in the fabric of our wishes, hopes, and dreams. Why are we drawn to one another? How does this relationship affect my life? What is God- or Goddess-like in our sexual union? What do I have to learn from being with my partner? From this broad perspective, we can view all of our relationships as sacred. Even an abusive relationship can be sacred, for once we open our eyes we find ourselves on a path of discovery. And then a major question is, "How long do I need to stay in this relationship to learn what I need to know?"

"Sacred Marriage"
Our Lineage of Power

At this point in our story of sacred sexual union, I ask us to look back into the past—because understanding where we came from can help us locate where we are and move us forward to where we want to go. Although connecting sex and spirit may be a new idea for many twenty-first-century Westerners, it's actually an old and fundamental idea in the sweep of human history. Cultural anthropologists have shown that sex and spirit, body and soul, were all considered intrinsic to one another way before the rise of the performance scripts so many of us set our clocks by today. This idea is rooted in the ancient concept of sacred marriage.

The basic belief behind sacred marriage is that the universe is born of divine beings. Images of cosmic matings appear in artifacts from every continent, and they date from as far back as Paleolithic times (30,000 to 12,000 B.C.E.). If you look through history, you can find a pantheon of randy gods and goddesses letting their libidos run free as they procreate earth, seas, sun, moon, stars, and human beings, too. There's Ishtar and Tammuz in Mesopotamia. There's Shakti and Shiva in India. There's Changing Woman and her consort, the Sun, among the North American Navaho Diné. The list goes on.

An abiding theme in all these creation stories is the sexual power of women. Female divinities were co-creators with male divinities. They possessed the ability to love, nurture, play, seduce and also destroy—no modern-day Mars-Venus inequalities here. These female deities were vortexes of sexual energy. For the mortals who hunted and tilled for a living, they modeled a luscious freewheeling brand of sexual desire—no 43 percent were branded dysfunctional the way today's women are by researchers who reduce sexual experience to activities they can count and measure.

Did you ever aspire to be a sex goddess? Well, it may require more than just getting a spa makeover and learning how to walk in high heels without toppling over. Here's what Oshun says—she's the Yoruban goddess of love, intimacy, beauty, and wealth: "Let me seduce you with scents, let me tantalize your taste till your tongue quivers, let me touch your body with waterfall music." When you consider all you might put yourself through for one wild and glorious night of love, why not go all the way to the source. Think, *"What would Isis do?"*

In ancient Egypt, Isis was known as the "goddess of a thousand names," including Initiator into the Sexual Mysteries. Her story goes that she circled the globe to search out the scattered parts of her husband Osiris, whose evil brother had hacked him into thirteen pieces. Isis was able to reconstitute him—but she couldn't locate his penis, which had been thrown into the Nile River and swallowed by a fish. Undaunted, she constructed a new penis out of Egyptian clay, then mounted Osiris to conceive their son— Horus of the all-seeing eye. You can call on Isis whenever the time comes to take sexual matters into your own hands. I have enduring personal gratitude for Isis, who appeared just when I needed an acronym for my survey, "Integrating Sexuality and Spirituality"—"ISIS"—voilà!

Another goddess with awesome sexual energy is Inanna. We met her in the previous chapter—the Sumerian version of the Great Mother, queen of the sky, goddess of fertility, and also the creator of the earliest love poem on record, "Inanna's Hymn." She addresses this song to Dumuzi, her consort, her "honey man." You can see from the fragment below that it expresses her divine sexual desire in earthy terms—and it foreshadows the lush sensual images in the biblical Song of Solomon, which wasn't to be written until some two thousand years later.

Fragment from Inanna's Hymn

He has sprouted; he has burgeoned;
He is lettuce planted by the water.
He is the one my womb loves best.

These exuberant gods and goddesses generated a significant trickle-down of attitudes to human beings—"as above, so below," say the old sages. When you look at cave paintings and early sculptures, it's evident that for most of human history erotic desire and pleasure were seen as a natural part of living. Sexual behavior wasn't always dictated by church or state. And it wasn't hidden behind closed doors. Sex was essential for creating life itself, and it was out there for all to see—and enjoy.

Sex was openly celebrated in religious worship, too, and centuries of repression haven't been able to purge it from our holy days and everyday altars. Vestiges remain, even in our major religions. Think flowers, wine, music, and dancing. Think laying on of hands, anointing with oil, words of love, and raising a joyful noise. All of these still play a part in religious ceremony. They still also play a part in sexual romance, of course. When you bring flowers to your sweetie or dance together or whisper sweet nothings or give each other loving back rubs and belly rubs, you're engaging in some level of sacred ceremony whether you're consciously aware of it or not.

Sacred Marriage Today
Our Power in the Now

Let's fast-forward to the present: I've heard many women report their own versions of sacred marriage. They speak eloquently of how connecting sex and spirit generates sexual desire. One woman praises her lover in phrases that link her with sacred lovers of history as surely as if she's a direct descendant of the early goddess traditions.

> He has allowed me the love (as unconditional as love can be for humans) to revere what is sacred, what is Godlike within myself, within himself, and in our lovemaking. Through his subtle encouragement, the environment I have placed myself in, and the personal work that I am doing, I have finally realized fully what it means to bring my spirituality and my sexuality together.

Like so many women I've seen in my practice, the road to this woman's present relationship was fraught with experiences that dammed up her flow of sexual desire—until she was almost thirty. She's a survivor of parental shaming, of a rocky sexual adolescence, and of a rape that resulted in a pregnancy she tried to abort. What reignited desire for her began with therapy and intense soul searching—which she says led her to the divine guidance that enabled her to tap into her own sexual wisdom. She woke up—in every sense and attitude. She started noticing the world around her. She stopped inviting destructive relationships. She began a new sexual partnership that felt sacred to her. And she developed a professional career as a massage therapist and healer that taught her respect for her body and "reverence for the sacredness that lies within each person."

> I am now in a space that allows me to celebrate my womanhood, my sexuality, and my spirituality together, without fear of being judged or being labeled or feeling the need to act out sexually in what was my own dysfunction. I have stopped judging myself, which allows me to have more inner peace, and that allows me more freedom to connect with God and vice versa.

Other women speak of sexual desire as a direct path to God, Goddess, and even Christ-as-bridegroom. For one wide-open woman it was a sudden and vibrant image that conveyed to her the magic of a sexual encounter with the divine.

> I felt as though a force field had been broken through. There was no pain; it felt as though my lover and I were going into new territory. When I opened my eyes to look at him, he looked like so many of the images we use for Jesus Christ. I stared in awe and wavering belief; he looked back with such compassion and understanding. I knew I had experienced knowing the Divine in my Beloved.

She says this encounter amazed her. It amazed her doubly because of its Christian imagery, as she'd abandoned her Christian beliefs and practices years before.

Her story is part of the living proof that the idea of sacred marriage wasn't lost when the world transitioned from those randy gods and goddesses to a monolithic asexual male, be that Jahweh, Allah, Buddha, or an omniscient "Father who art in heaven." Christian history (for one) boasts a lineage of love mystics, who experienced Christ as more than just a disembodied spirit. He was also their personal lover and bridegroom. My onetime favorite love mystic is Teresa of Ávila, the sixteenth-century nun who maintained astounding records of her orgasmic "raptures" with Christ and his flame-bearing angels. She writes that these experiences struck her speechless with awe, but her *Vida* runs to some 560 pages. Bernini's celebrated statue in the basilica of Santa Maria Della Vittoria in Rome shows Saint Teresa in mid-ecstasy, eyes rolled back, the skirts of her habit rumpled as the sheets of a marriage bed.

The notion of sacred union may be age-old—but it speaks to our hunger for more connectedness and meaning in our sexual relationships today. It speaks to the brilliance and resilience of our twenty-first-century longings as we seek to move more fully into the space capsules we call our bodies and into our sensual, sexual selves. It speaks to the return of sexual desire—not as a pharmaceutically induced phenomenon, but as a gift to and from our bodies, minds, hearts, and souls.

Four Sacred Questions

Here are four questions that women say help open their eyes, ears, hearts, and bodies to the notion of sacred union. These questions can profoundly affect your opening up to sexual desire—because answering them honestly can bring home how the sacred is everywhere in our experience of pleasure, sometimes in the simplest physical activities. I've heard these questions used by spiritual teachers as a way of determining one's readiness to enter the realm of spirit. They're all about how willing you are to make time to open up and feel.

When did you last dance?

When did you last sing?

When did you last spend quality time alone with yourself?

When did you last tell your story?

You can ask these questions of yourself. Some people find that simply reading the questions is enough to create a shift of consciousness and intention for their lives. If you want to explore these questions further, answer them from all your perspectives—body, mind, heart, and spirit. I love what author Byron Katie (*A Thousand Names for Joy*) says about tapping into your inner wisdom so that you reach beyond just your mental capacity: "Ask, then be still and wait for an inner voice to respond. With practice, this will become easier. You will learn to rely on yourself—not the world—to see what's true for you."

You can do this exercise with your partner, too, by asking the four questions of each other. Try asking them all at once and listen to your partner's response. Allow at least five minutes for your partner to respond. Be sure to turn off your TV and cell phones, and take any other steps that ensure your privacy.

Five minutes can seem like a eternity for some and not nearly long enough for others. However it seems for you, just listen in open attention, without offering suggestions or trying to edit what your partner says. It's OK if there's some silence. As Katie suggests, silence doesn't necessarily mean nothing's happening. Some of the great shifts of consciousness have occurred in silence—think Newton and the apple, think Jesus in the desert.

Once your partner has spoken to these questions, trade roles so your partner does the asking and listening.

Some partners find it helps to repeat the Q and A process several times. This gives you an opportunity to reach deeper inside yourselves for layers of meaning you may not get to on the first go-round. On your final round it can be valuable to phrase these questions in the form of a commitment: "When (and how) *will* you next dance/sing/spend quality time alone/tell your story?"

And if it works for you, try a round that phrases these questions as invitations to play: "Let's dance together/sing together/spend quality time together/tell our stories to each other."

However you decide to engage with these questions, the spirit behind them is to encourage answers that come from the heart—especially for the question about telling your own story. This is a perfect lead-in for telling your new story about sexual desire—which will be the subject of the final chapter of this book. Allow plenty of time. And be open to the outcome.

Your Inner Journey to Sacred Pleasure

The technique of visualization is a time-honored way to access insights and feelings you may not notice on an everyday basis. A childbirth educator who attended one of my workshops described her process of visualization as an inner journey—like logging on to a richly informational website with constantly new and fascinating data. She shared with us that she'd uncovered a ravenous Inner Panther—a cross between a sacred power animal and a sex-crazed goddess—and she was looking forward to visiting with her again and again and again.

Below is a guided visualization to help you open up to pleasure, and to the sacredness of pleasure. You can benefit from this visualization even if you have no previous experience with visualization or meditation. In addition to reading it on the page, I invite you to ask someone to read it to you while you allow yourself to meditate and "journey." Or you can record it and play it back to yourself. It takes about eight minutes to read aloud.

Consider sharing this inner journey with your partner. After you've each completed your trip, you have an opportunity to talk about where it led you—perhaps to a depth of feeling and desire that may be new. This kind of conversation may stimulate you to create your new story about sexual desire—Inner Panthers and all. Your sharing may bypass words entirely and lead from opening your hearts and minds to exploring each other's bodies.

When I offer this kind of visualization in workshops, the sharing becomes rich in a quantum way—as if there's a leap of understanding for the entire group. The resonance is often strong enough to reach women who've never been able to experience how sexual energy can be spiritual as well as physical.

So get yourself in a comfortable position, kick back, and open to the experience—whether it turns out to be quantum or not.

Opening Your Heart and Mind to Sacred Pleasure
A Guided Visualization

Close your eyes. Slowly take a deep breath—in—and slowly let it all the way out. If you find any places in your being that are holding tension, breathe softly into them and give them permission to let go and relax. That includes your belief system. Allow all the muscles and psychic muscles that hold your beliefs together to let out a big sigh and relax for a while.

Your breath is what connects you to yourself—body, mind, heart, and spirit. So take a moment to be aware of how your breath travels constantly through your whole being—and your whole life.

Imagine that you can follow your breath back in time—to a time when you remember feeling deep pleasure. The kind that makes you smile whenever you think about it.

Perhaps this was very recently. Or maybe it was way back when you were a kid—splashing in water, snuggling with a pet, or discovering that you could ride a bike. Remember how good you felt. Where do you notice this feeling in your body now? Remember how powerful you felt—not the kind of power that wants to dominate other people, but the kind of power that wants to share. Feel that power now and breathe it into your body, your mind, your heart, and your spirit.

Allow this feeling of pleasure and power to surround you now—like sunshine or the soft breath of an evening breeze. Be aware of moving around now in a whole landscape of pleasure and pulsating power. How big is the space? Who's there? Who's not there? What does it feel like to let yourself be in this place of pleasure and power? Be aware of your breathing—as you continue to breathe in . . . and out.

And now follow your breath to the very center of your being—your own heart.

Feel your heart gently expanding.

Breathe into that expansion.

And now breathe that expansion down through your body—through your belly, through your pelvis, through your genitals, through your thighs, calves, feet, all the way into the ground, deep down into the earth. And breathe it back up again—through your feet and legs and genitals and pelvis and belly—all the way up to your heart again.

And now, breathe that expansion from your heart up through your throat and all the way up to the top of your head—as if you could open up the crown of your head and expand yourself way up into the heavens. Into the luminosity of the sun and the moon and the stars.

And breathe all that light back in and let it shine into your mind. Let it illuminate everything it touches.

As you look around in your luminous mind, you notice that there's a message waiting for you. This message has your name on it. See this message now. Or hear it. Or feel it. This is a message about pleasure. About physical pleasure. About sexual pleasure. About the holiness of pleasure and desire. About what *you* need *more* of in your life *now*.

Very clearly now, be aware of this message. On your next breath you're going to deliver it straight to your heart. From your mind to your heart. Special delivery.

Feel what it's like when both your heart and your mind experience this message about the holiness of feeling good.

Breathe it in and experience whatever is true for you . . .

And when you're ready, prepare yourself to bring your new knowledge back to the here and now—to your life. Thank your heart. Thank your mind. Thank your body. Thank your breath for leading you on this journey.

As you begin to wiggle your fingers and toes and come back to the present—know in your deepest soul that you can open your heart and mind to pleasure whenever you want. All you have to do is breathe . . .

Welcome home . . . to *yourself*.

13

WHAT WOMEN WANT
Expanding Your Own Story of Sexual Desire

THE ROUTE to great sex is like the route to any other of life's deep mysteries. It means exploring new emotional landscapes. It means opening your wild, precious, vulnerable self and allowing the Divine to move through your body. It means daring to know what you want.

What do you want? How do you plan to ask for it? What will you do with it once it comes to you? Throughout this book, you've read stories culled from experiences of thousands of other women—and hundreds of men. Now it's time for you to speak for yourself—perhaps to expand the story of your own sexual desire beyond what you once believed were the absolute limits.

There's the popular myth that desire ought to be spontaneous, a kind of hormonal *deus ex machina* that drops from the heavens while you're folding the laundry. But for many of us desire takes conscious preparation. Even contemplating what you might want can take preparation—especially if you've been raised to believe that good girls *don't*, and aren't supposed to speak up about it, either. Think of Cleopatra and her triumphal entry into Rome. The elephants, the jugglers, the plumed canopy. What kind of procession do you need for your sexual desire to blossom and flower?

I'm an eternal optimist, and I believe your life will be better when you can answer these questions—even if they are difficult for you. I believe that answering these questions will make your life better even if you have a sexual partner who can already play you like a magic flute. And I believe that becoming clear about all the aspects of what you want and what you don't want will also make your life better even if you don't have a partner. Because at the end of the day, the being who most needs to hear this information is *you*.

Find the Space to Explore
A Honeymoon of One's Own

As you've read in every chapter of this book, opening up to all the energies of sexual desire means more than just activating the requisite hormones and neurotransmitters. It also means expanding our whole lives and nourishing our spirits. A word I hear again and again from women is "connection." We crave a sense of oneness with our partners, ourselves, and the universe. We yearn for touch and love and meaning. And we long for these even though we may be embarrassed or scared, or reeling from histories of hurt and disappointment.

But not all of us want to be immersed totally in our partners, not for long anyway. Even in the closest relationships, we need some downtime, some space to be ourselves. Feminist novelist Virginia Woolf famously wrote of the need for "a room of one's own." She uses this phrase in reference to British women in the 1920s, but it speaks volumes about our current requirements for the return of sexual desire into our lives—the need for privacy, for time out from housework, child care, aging parents, and on and on.

You may need a room of your own to provide the space for you to recognize your deepest sexual desires. And if you can't afford the actual real estate, you may need to create some kind of psychic and emotional space all for yourself. I'm not talking just about scheduling a haircut or massage, indulgent as that may seem. I mean making the space to think and feel and connect with your own inner being.

A friend who was about to embark on a honeymoon with her second husband echoed this sentiment when she confided, "He asked me where I wanted to go, and all I could think of was how wonderful it would be to just go someplace all by myself where I could regroup and reenergize." It wasn't that she didn't care for her new husband—or that she didn't look forward to some hot honeymoon loving. Her statement sprang from her need to recover her own identity, amid the chaos of amalgamating two boisterous families—five children, two dogs, various parents, stepparents, grandparents, and more.

Her idea made so much sense to me that I routinely suggest women take themselves on solo honeymoons every once in a while—to refresh their senses and spirits, to connect with themselves, to be still and listen. If you can afford a pricey spa vacation, well and good. But you can also keep it simple. How about an afternoon by a rippling stream? How about a date with your journal, or your favorite music, or your trusty vibrator? An hour or even ten minutes stolen from a hectic day can help rejuvenate you. Meditate. Smell a flower. Take a shower. Take a walk. Take a nap. Or just breathe. Often it's in our breathing that we find the space to visualize what we want—to feel it in our bodies, know it in our minds, hearts, and spirits.

Follow Your Dreams

It's crucial to understand the difference between your fantasies and your deepest dreams. Fantasies offer delicious hassle-free vacations from your everyday activities. You can be Sleeping Beauty, Sex Goddess, Queen for a Day. Your fantasies can refresh and restore you. They can inform your sexual desire, but they may not be reliable to hitch your wagon to. As one woman admits of her forays into her fantasy world of bondage with rock stars, "They're great places to visit, but I wouldn't want to live there."

A dream is your heart's desire—that comes from deep within you and that motivates you, body, mind, heart, and spirit. "To hell with happiness—I want ecstasy!" This is how a beloved colleague expressed her sexual dream to me many years ago. I find myself weaving her into book after book because her spirit brings me so much joy—the kind that calls out to be shared. Her exclamation urges us to think big, to refuse to settle for a life that's half-full.

What is your dream? Your happiness? Your ecstasy? Many of us discover the answers bubbling up through the actual dreams that come to us in sleep—the level of consciousness that slips under the radar of cultural conditioning. Images and stories revealed here can be powerful guides to what we want and the sexual directions we want to follow.

Here's how one woman began to explore a crucial question in her sexual story—whether or not to commit to a new relationship with an old flame. She'd come to one of my workshops with her college-student daughter, which I think was bravely adventurous of both of them. I tell her story as an example of how the universe can help you clarify what you want if only you stop, look, and listen.

A week after the workshop, this woman had a dream that shifted her fear of commitment and opened her to exploring a new level of sexual desire. In the dream, she was confronted by a huge lion whose mane was braided with golden bells. On the one hand, she was terrified by the lion—she feared it was going to tear her apart and kill her. On the other hand, she was elated, because she also recognized the lion as a protector, a benevolent being from the spirit world who was sent to deliver a message that would change her view of life and death—and give new direction to the form her sexual desire might take.

Later, as she reflected on the dream, she understood that part of the lion's message was indeed about her death. But it was not about her physical death. It was about tearing apart and killing off the fear that no longer served her—especially the fear of fully engaging in the new sexual relationship with her old love. It was as if her dream was revealing a process of healing and transformation, the kind that can take place instantly and magically. She ultimately accepted the dream as a kind of shamanic initiation—in which the spirits dismember the old dysfunctional you, then put you back together, more completely whole and with a new lease on personal power. In her case the new lease on power was permission to allow herself to feel the full range of her desire to join her new relationship—and at this writing she says she's committed to doing exactly that.

Not all of us can conjure up such a magical dream to help guide how we'll follow our wild and precious desires. But we can all use our imaginations. When you're rescripting your own story, remember to factor in all your experiences of sexual desire including your daydreams and nightdreams. Prepare to expect the unexpected. The basic lesson here is that sexual desire has many faces—and the major one belongs to *you*.

Make It Tangible

I've found that the more concretely you can allow yourself to think about what you want, the more easily a new story can unfold for you. A question I routinely ask women who come to my workshops is: What parts of your sexual story do you want to keep—what parts do you want to nurture and build on?

Think about an object that would represent the most positive and hopeful aspects of *your* sexual story—something to remind you of what you want to manifest in your life. This object might be a crystal, a flower, a picture, a book. Maybe it's a wedding ring or a commitment ring. Maybe it's a mirror to represent your acceptance of your body and your self. Maybe it's a candle to represent the ongoing flame of your sexual desire. Maybe it's a piece of fabric to represent the warmth and color of your capacity for love. Maybe it's a yardstick or a map to show how far you've come on your path. Maybe it's a musical instrument. One woman said she wanted to invoke a full orchestra to represent what she felt when she experienced her first orgasm—at age forty-eight.

What kind of object comes to mind as you think about your positive sexual story? What part of your story does it represent for you? What does it say about your sexual desire? What's it like for you to put your experience of sexual desire into such a concrete form or image?

Sometimes an object presents itself immediately. But don't worry if you have to search around until the right piece appears. It doesn't have to be perfect. And it doesn't have to be forever. Over time, you may find many objects that represent many positive aspects of your story. Sometimes you can actively choose your object. Sometimes your object seems to reach out and choose you.

Another workshop participant said she'd kept searching for something in nature that would represent steadfast loyalty, which was the quality she most admired in her own sexual story—but she felt flummoxed, because she couldn't seem to find an object that was just right. Besides, each time she walked around her yard, she stubbed her toe on a big rock that jutted into her path. "Ouch!" She finally got it that this rock was calling out to her, "I'm here!" So she picked it up—and understood that this was exactly it—*steady as a rock.*

So take whatever time you need to find your object—and notice your journey. Once you've found what feels right, hold it, and visualize the feelings you want it to represent. Close your eyes and breathe these feelings into your heart so you can taste them and smell them and sense their texture. Now, with soft breath blow all those feelings into your object—as if you can literally breathe life into it. Feel the warmth that floods into your hand.

By breathing your object into life, you have created a medicine piece—a healing tool that radiates positive energy. As you keep it in your consciousness, it will help you attract more positive energy, more desire. And it will help you clear away any dense, negative energy that creeps back into your sexuality or your life.

Find a special place for your new medicine piece—on an altar if you have one, or in a window you love because you love the view. This object represents a memory, a feeling, a wish, a meaningful part of your sexual story you want to keep. Give it a good home. Pay attention to it. Gaze at it. Talk to it. Hold it. Bring it flowers. Treat it like a lover. I'm not asking you to be weird. Just to pay attention.

Create a Manifesto for Sexual Desire

Now it's time for you to move beyond this book to write your own story, your own manifesto. Let it come from your heart. You can write it as a love letter to yourself. Or you can address it as a love letter to your partner—or to the partner you wish you had. Why not make it delicious enough to keep under your pillow to evoke erotic dreams on a regular basis?

What will you ask for? There can be enormous variation in what you want and what other women may want—dress-up? bubble baths? oral sex? anal stimulation? having your wrists lashed to the bedpost with red silk pantyhose? One woman's sexual desire may be another's big yawn. Or big yuck. And what you wanted with a former lover may be very different from your greatest joy with your present partner. And what you wanted at age twenty-one may be light-years away from what makes your heart leap and your spine tingle at age forty-six, or seventy-two.

Below is a compilation of some of the desires I've heard from women whose stories are in this book. I call it "Lessons from Women Who Love Sex"— borrowed from the title of my earlier book, to honor all the unnamed women who've opened their hearts to me over the years. Let this compilation be your guide if it resonates with you. But don't let it inhibit your creativity. I include it to show some of the breadth—and contradictions—of women's sexual desire. Mostly, I include it to encourage you to be as open as you can about listing all that you want for *you*. So have a look. See which ones work for you, and which ones don't. Above all, add your own specifics as you compile the shopping list for your own journey to the return of desire. (You can find a color poster of this manifesto on my website: www.GinaOgden.com.)

When Good Girls Do
LESSONS FROM *WOMEN WHO LOVE SEX*

women want honesty . women want to feel good . women want to let go . women want information . women want respect . women want to open their hearts . women want to dance . women want to make love on the hood of a car . women want a soulmate . women want to turn their lives around . women want foreplay . women want fairplay . women want love . women want to be noticed . women want flowers . women want men to stop asking dumb questions . women want closeness . women want space for themselves . women want to expand their vision . women want vibrators . women want to play . women want to find themselves . women want safety . women want to be vulnerable . women want women . women want to revel in new love . women want to be courted . women want clitoral stimulation . women want self-esteem . women want nurturing . women want power . women want to share . women want pleasure . women want orgasms . women want mystery . women want kink . women want someone else to do the dishes . women want to be transported beyond themselves . women want dirty dancing . women want more than one lover . women want one faithful sexual partner their whole lives long . women want to be touched all over . women want to dress up . women want right relationship . women want sweetness . women want loyalty . women want to swim naked . women want to be heard . women want you to pay attention . women want to be recognized as the goddesses they are

---

AFTERWORD

Like Fine Wine—When Desire Ripens with Age

AT LAST, the billion-dollar question: what happens to sexual desire as we grow older? The prevailing notion is that it goes downhill from the instant you spot your first gray hair. You know the drill. First your looks collapse. Then your self-esteem. Your pubic hair thins, you cease to lubricate lushly, your relationship falls apart, and you fade slowly into your sunset years watching TV reality shows and munching bags of Cheetos.

In this scenario, it's as if all women of a certain age are doomed to stop responding to the present and become dusty archives of past loves, past lives. Indeed, this is the story for some women. And this is good news for the pharmaceutical companies, as it helps them sell their products—the so-called horny pills, creams, and patches. In fact pharmaceutical companies regularly commission the medical research that says we need these products if we're ever going to feel our sexual oats again. With an estimated 70 million baby-boomer women entering midlife and beyond within the next few years, dare I suggest that we boomers—and post-boomers—can think of ourselves as veritable cash cows.

But take heart. This doesn't have to be your story. As we've seen throughout this book, there are other scenarios of sex and aging that may unfold. A major premise of *The Return of Desire* is that sexual experience is multidimensional and that individual differences reign supreme. News flash! Our sexual energy continues to be multidimensional and individual as we age, too. No one approach fits us all. No one prescription fits us all, either.

Certainly, there are changes in our desire over the years. But they're not always the changes we've been warned about—and this is a well-kept secret. The truth is, sexual desire and satisfaction do not have to go downhill with age. For some of us they can reach new heights. When we connect sexual desire with our emotional feelings and with what our intimate relationships mean to our lives, our sexual satisfaction may increase with every decade—say thousands of women who answered my ISIS survey. Most of the fifty-, sixty-, and seventy-year-olds in that sample were having a better time than the twenty- and thirty-year-olds.

These women say that sex can become less frenetic and goal driven as they grow older. And they say their sexual relationships can become more meaningful, more connected, more whole. These women describe moving beyond the shoulds and oughts that held them hostage when they were younger—from good-girl constraints to good-wife partner-pleasing. Some of them say that through the years they've been able to shake blissfully free of the devastating legacy of abuse and violence that's haunted them from girlhood.

My gratitude forever to the respondents of the ISIS survey, all 3,810 of them. Their collective wisdom is that desire means more than an increasing dependence on pharmaceuticals. And that it means more than just growing up and shucking the negatives out of our lives. For some, it takes conscious cultivation of self-esteem—sexual confidence and fullness of expression. And these are qualities that life experience may enhance rather than erode away. Christiane Northrup is eloquent on this subject in her book *The Wisdom of Menopause,* where she describes the optimism and uppitiness that can keep women blooming well-nigh forever.

This late-blooming self-esteem carries over into our relationships with our lovers. Some women who've lived on this planet for a long time have been able to tap into extraordinary depths of relational richness. For them, age seems to usher in a process of transformation—as if our sexual beings can actually mature and ripen, like fine wine.

What a radical way to think about sex and aging.

What about those hormones and pills? Some women thrive on them, some don't. Keep an open mind about the aphrodisiac quality of commercial products. For some women there's much to be said for a rush of dopamine, a spurt of oxytocin, a dash of testosterone or estrogen. And be aware that you may be able to get these aphrodisiac effects without using products. The truth is, self-esteem and intimacy and erotic touching ultimately produce the same physiological rush.

Notice how the whole sexual picture becomes brighter for women when we think about sexual aging in terms of feelings and meanings instead of frequencies of sexual intercourse. For some of us, it's as if we've been blown out of Kansas and into Oz. A woman in her late fifties describes how her desire keeps expanding with her long-term partner.

> The love of my husband during sex just grew and grew until the actual hairs on his body sparkled. He became so beautiful and has remained that way.

Among my favorite ISIS survey respondents is a couple who answered the survey together—as one voice. They state their age as "seventy-four years young," and their occupation as "sexually active." Their sexual intimacy has evolved over their long life together, and includes a broad gamut, from earthy and physical to universal and divine. Their eloquence speaks for itself.

> The bottom line to this letter is that oneness in love is a prolonged time of at least four to six hours of foreplay, oral sex (whatever pleases the other), culminating in spiritual orgasm simultaneously where for a sacred moment the bodies blend as one, and the face of creation is seen. There is more that can be said and we are more than willing to be interviewed with the exposure of our names.

What I love most about this quote is the openness it radiates. And its ringing optimism. I offer it here as inspiration—as long as you don't take it as some kind of standard you have to shoot for by the time you reach seventy-four. Sexual desire can flourish even if you never make love for six hours without stopping or get to see the "face of creation."

Life changes. Bodies change. Sexual desire changes. But there's no one right way to feel sexual desire, to express our sexuality, or to grow older. Only you can say what all the changes are and what they mean for you.

How women experience these changes in their sexual stories will be the focus of my next book—*The Best Is Yet to Come: Women Talk about Love, Sex, and Aging*. It will include breaking news, such as findings from the AARP survey on sex and aging and advice from the anti-aging front—a whole new specialty field of medicine. But mainly it will focus on women—our feelings, our stories, our unique wisdom.

Meanwhile, may you continue to reach out for loving contact. May you never lose the hunger for feeling good.

The Extragenital Matrix: sexual enjoyment beyond the usual "homing sites"

Rate from 0 to 10 (0-not all, 10-ecstatic) how much you enjoy various kinds of touch on different parts of your body

Kinds of Touch
TOUCHING BY HAND

WHERE ON MY BODY	Soft Stroking	Deep Stroking	Rubbing	Patting	
Head and Face					
Hair/scalp					
Cheeks					
Lips					
Ears					
Neck and Torso					
Neck					
Shoulders					
Stomach					
Back					
Buttocks					
Arms and Hands					
Arms					
Elbows					
Wrists					
Palms					
Fingers					
Legs and Feet					
Legs					
Ankles					
Feet					
Toes					
Full Body					
Other					

KINDS OF TOUCH
TOUCHING BY MOUTH

Kissing	Licking	Sucking	Nipping	WHERE ON MY BODY
				Head and Face
				Hair/scalp
				Cheeks
				Lips
				Ears
				Neck and Torso
				Neck
				Shoulders
				Stomach
				Back
				Buttocks
				Arms and Hands
				Arms
				Elbows
				Wrists
				Palms
				Fingers
				Legs and Feet
				Legs
				Ankles
				Feet
				Toes
				Full Body
				Other

SUGGESTED READINGS
(AND VIEWINGS)

Understanding the Intelligence of Our Bodies

BOOKS

Angier, Natalie. *Woman: An Intimate Geography.* Boston: Houghton Mifflin, 1999.

Blank, Joani. *Femalia.* San Francisco: Down There Press, 1993.

Boston Women's Health Book Collective. *Our Bodies, Ourselves: A New Edition for a New Era.* Rev. ed. New York: Simon and Schuster, 2005.

Buss, David. *The Evolution of Desire: Strategies of Human Mating.* New York: Basic Books, 2003.

Camphause, Rufus. *The Yoni: Sacred Symbol of Female Creative Power.* Rochester, Vt.: Inner Traditions, 1996.

Chalker, Rebecca. *The Clitoral Truth: The Secret World at Our Fingertips.* New York: Seven Stories Press, 2000.

Conrad, Emilie. *Life on Land: The Story of Continuum.* Berkeley, Calif.: North Atlantic Books, 2007.

Dodson, Betty. *Sex for One: The Joy of Self-Loving.* Rev. ed. New York: Crown, 1996.

Giddings, Paula. *When and Where I Enter: The Impact of Black Women on Race and Sex in America.* New York: William Morrow, 1984.

Karras, Nick. *Petals.* San Diego, Calif.: Crystal River Publishing, 2003.

Maltz, Wendy, and Suzie Boss. *Private Thoughts: Exploring the Power of Women's Sexual Fantasies.* New York: New World Library, 2001.

Miller, Marshall, and Dorian Solat. *I Love Female Orgasm.* New York: Marlowe and Company, 2007.

Northrup, Christiane. *Women's Bodies, Women's Wisdom: Creating Physical and Emotional Health and Healing.* New York: Bantam, 1995.

Tisdale, Sallie. *Talk Dirty to Me: An Intimate Philosophy of Sex.* New York: Anchor, 1995.

DVDs

Dodson, Betty. *Selfloving: Portrait of a Women's Sexuality Seminar.* DVD. Pacific Media, 2005.

Slick, Wendy, and Emiko Omori, directors. *Passion and Power: The Technology of Orgasm.* San Francisco: Wabi Sabi Productions, 2007.

Creating Right Sexual Relationship with Ourselves and Our Partners

BOOKS

Anapol, Deborah. *Polyamory: The New Love without Limits: Secrets of Sustainable Intimate Relationships.* Rev. ed. San Raphael, Calif.: IntiNet Resource Center, 1997.

Britton, Patti. *The Art of Sex Coaching: Expanding Your Practice.* New York: W. W. Norton, 2005.

Suggested Readings (and Viewings)

Cambridge Women's Pornography Cooperative. *Porn for Women.* New York: Chronicle, 2007.

Castleman, Michael. *Great Sex: A Man's Guide to the Secret Principles of Total-Body Sex.* New York: Rodale, 2004.

Coontz, Stephanie. *Marriage, a History: From Obedience to Intimacy, or, How Love Conquered Marriage.* New York: Viking, 2005.

Cornog, Martha. *The Big Book of Masturbation: From Angst to Zeal.* San Francisco: Down There Press, 2003.

Eason, Dossie, and Catherine Liszt. *The Ethical Slut: A Guide to Infinite Sexual Possibilities.* Oakland, Calif.: Greenery Press, 1998.

Eisler, Riane. *The Power of Partnership: Seven Relationships That Will Change Your Life.* New York: New World Library, 2002.

Ensler, Eve. *The Vagina Monologues: The V-Day Edition.* New York: Villard, 2000.

Foley, Sallie, Sally Kope, and Dennis Sugrue. *Sex Matters for Women: A Complete Guide to Taking Care of Your Sexual Self.* Binghamton, N.Y.: Guilford Press, 2002.

Francoeur, Robert T., Martha Cornog, and Timothy Perper, eds. *Sex, Love, and Marriage in the Twenty-first Century: The Next Sexual Revolution.* Lincoln, Neb.: iUniverse.com, 1999.

Hall, Kathryn. *Reclaiming Your Sexual Self: How You Can Bring Desire Back into Your Life.* Hoboken, N.J.: Wiley, 2004.

Joannides, Paul. *Guide to Getting It On.* 5th ed. Waldport, Ore.: Goofy Foot Press, 2006.

Kerner, Ian. *She Comes First: The Thinking Man's Guide to Pleasuring a Woman.* New York: Regan Books, 2004.

Lerner, Harriet Goldhor. *The Dance of Anger: A Woman's Guide to Changing the Patterns of Intimate Relationships.* New York: Harper & Row, 1986.

———. *The Dance of Intimacy: A Woman's Guide to Courageous Acts of Change in Key Relationships.* New York: Harper & Row, 1989.

Loe, Meika. *The Rise of Viagra: How the Little Blue Pill Changed Sex in America.* New York: New York University Press, 2004.

Ogden, Gina. *Women Who Love Sex: Ordinary Women Describe Their Paths to Pleasure, Intimacy, and Ecstasy.* Rev. ed. Boston: Shambhala/Trumpeter, 2007.

Perel, Esther. *Mating in Captivity: Reconciling the Erotic and the Domestic.* New York: HarperCollins, 2006.

Real, Terrence. *The New Rules of Marriage: What You Need to Know to Make Love Work.* New York: Ballantine, 2007.

Resnick, Stella. *The Pleasure Zone: How to Let Go of Control and Be Happy.* Los Angeles: Conari Press, 1997.

Sprinkle, Annie. *Dr. Sprinkle's Spectacular Sex: Make Over Your Love Life with One of the World's Great Sex Experts.* New York: Jeremy Tarcher, 2005.

DVDs

Eastwood, Clint, director. *The Bridges of Madison County.* 1995. DVD. Warner Home Video, 1997.

Ferran, Pascale, director. *Lady Chatterley.* DVD. Kino Video, 2007.

Jhally, Sut, director. *Killing Us Softly 3: Advertising's Image of Women.* DVD. Media Education Foundation, 2000.

Creating Sacred Sexual Union

BOOKS

Allione, Tsultrim. *Women of Wisdom.* London: Routledge and Kegan Paul, 1984.

Anand, Margo. *The Art of Sexual Ecstasy: The Path of Sacred Sexuality for Western Lovers.* Los Angeles: Jeremy Tarcher, 1989.

Beattie-Jung, Patricia, Mary E. Hunt, and Radhika Balakrishnan. *Good Sex: Feminist Perspectives from the World's Religions.* New Brunswick, N.J.: Rutgers University Press, 2001.

Bonheim, Jalaja. *Aphrodite's Daughters: Women's Sexual Stories and the Journey of the Soul.* New York: Fireside, 1997.

Brock, Rita N. *Journeys by Heart: A Christology of Erotic Power.* New York: Crossroad, 1988.

Eisler, Riane. *Sacred Pleasure: Sex, Myth, and the Politics of the Body.* San Francisco: HarperCollins, 1995.

Gendreau, Geralyn, ed. *The Marriage of Sex and Spirit: Relationships at the Heart of Conscious Evolution.* Santa Rosa, Calif.: Elite Books, 2006.

Gimbutas, Marija. *The Language of the Goddess.* San Francisco: Harper & Row, 1989.

Guy, David. *The Red Thread of Passion: Spirituality and the Paradox of Sex.* Boston: Shambhala, 1999.

Heyward, Carter. *Touching Our Strength: The Erotic as Power and the Love of God.* New York: HarperCollins, 1989.

Hendricks, Gay. *Ecstatic Sex.* Audio CD. Louisville, Colo.: Sounds True, 2004.

Moore, Thomas. *The Soul of Sex: Cultivating Life as an Act of Love.* New York: HarperCollins, 1998.

Ogden, Gina. *The Heart and Soul of Sex: Making the ISIS Connection.* Boston: Trumpeter Books, 2006.

Savage, Linda E. *Reclaiming Goddess Sexuality: The Power of the Feminine Way.* Carlsbad, Calif.: Hay House, 1999.

Shaw, Miranda. *Passionate Enlightenment: Women in Tantric Buddhism.* Princeton, N.J.: Princeton University Press, 1994.

Somé, Sobonfu E. *The Spirit of Intimacy: Ancient Teachings in the Ways of Relationships.* Berkeley, Calif.: Berkeley Hills Books, 1997.

Stubbs, Kenneth Ray. *The Essential Tantra: A Modern Guide to Sacred Sexuality.* New York: Jeremy Tarcher, 1999.

Timmerman, Joan H. *Sexuality and Spiritual Growth.* New York: Crossroad, 1992.

Wade, Jenny. *Transcendent Sex: When Lovemaking Opens the Veil.* New York: Paraview Pocket Books, 2004.

Suggested Readings (and Viewings)

DVDs
Stubbs, Kenneth Ray, director. *Magdalene Unveiled: The Ancient and Modern Sacred Prostitute*. 2006. Tucson, Ariz.: Secret Garden Publishing, 2006.

Sex-Positive Birthing and Parenting
BOOKS
Boston Women's Health Book Collective. *Our Bodies Ourselves: Pregnancy and Birth*. New York: Touchstone, 2008.

Carroll, Janell. *Sexuality Now*. 2nd ed. Belmont, Calif.: Thomson, 2007.

Gaskin, Ina May. *Ina May's Guide to Childbirth*. New York: Bantam, 2001.

Haffner, Debra W. *From Diapers to Dating: A Parent's Guide to Raising Sexually Healthy Children—From Infancy to Middle School*. Rev. ed. New York: Newmarket Press, 2004.

Hamkins, SuEllen, and Renee Schultz. *The Mother-Daughter Project: How Mothers and Daughters Can Band Together, Beat the Odds, and Thrive through Adolescence*. New York: Hudson Street Press, 2007.

Harris, Robie, and Michael Emberley. *It's Perfectly Normal: Changing Bodies, Growing Up, Sex, and Sexual Health*. Rev. ed. Cambridge, Mass.: Candlewick Press, 2004.

Leboyer, Frederick. *Birth without Violence*. New York: Knopf, 1975.

Levine, Judith. *Harmful to Minors: The Perils of Protecting Children from Sex*. New York: Thundermouth Press, 2003.

Paget, Lou. *Hot Mamas: The Ultimate Guide to Staying Sexy throughout Your Pregnancy and the Months Beyond*. Scarborough, Ont.: Doubleday Canada, 2006.

Phipher, Mary. *Reviving Ophelia: Saving the Selves of Adolescent Girls*. New York: Ballantine, 1994.

Tolman, Deborah L. *Dilemmas of Desire: Teenage Girls Talk about Sexuality*. Cambridge, Mass.: Harvard University Press, 2003.

DVDs
Dayton, Jonathan, and Valerie Faris, directors. *Little Miss Sunshine*. 2006. DVD. Hollywood: Twentieth Century Fox, 2006.

Ridberg, Ronit, director. *Spin the Bottle: Sex, Lies, and Alcohol*. DVD. Media Education Foundation, 2004.

Letting Desire Out of the Cultural Box—Lesbian, Gay, Bisexual, and Transgender Relationships
BOOKS
Buxton, Amity P. *The Other Side of the Closet: The Coming-Out Crisis for Straight Spouses*. Santa Monica Calif.: IBS Press, 1991.

Eugenides, Jeffrey. *Middlesex*. New York: Farrar, Straus and Giroux, 2002.

Faderman, Lillian. *Surpassing the Love of Men: Romantic Friendship and Love between Women from the Renaissance to the Present*. New York: Morrow, 1981.

Feinberg, Leslie. *Transgender Warriors: Making History from Joan of Arc to RuPaul*. Boston: Beacon Press, 1997.

Graff, E. J. *What Is Marriage For?* Boston: Beacon Press, 1999.

Hall, Marny. *The Lesbian Love Companion*. San Francisco: Harper San Francisco, 1998.

Hoffman, Amy. *An Army of Ex-Lovers: My Life at Gay Community News*. Boston: University of Massachusetts Press, 2007.

Hutchins, Loraine, and Lani Kaahumanu, eds. *Bi Any Other Name: Bisexual People Speak Out*. Los Angeles: Alyson Publications, 1991.

DVDs

Edwards, Blake, director. *Victor Victoria*. 1982. DVD. Turner Home Video, 2002.

Lee, Ang, director. *Brokeback Mountain*. 2005. DVD. Hollywood: Universal, 2006.

Mitchell, John Cameron, director. *Shortbus*. 2006. DVD. Velocity/Think Film, 2007.

Nichols, Mike, director. *The Birdcage*. 1996. DVD. Hollywood: MGM, 1997.

Pollack, Sydney, director. *Tootsie*. 1982. DVD. Columbia Tri-Star, 2001.

Healing from Trauma—with Emotional and Sexual Integrity

BOOKS

Bass, Ellen, and Laura Davis. *The Courage to Heal: A Guide for Women Survivors of Child Sexual Abuse*. New York: Harper & Row, 1988.

Greenspan, Miriam. *Healing through the Dark Emotions: The Wisdom of Grief, Fear, and Despair*. Boston: Shambhala, 2004.

Haines, Staci. *The Survivor's Guide to Sex: How to Have an Empowered Sex Life after Child Sexual Abuse*. San Francisco: Cleis Press, 1999.

Herman, Judith Lewis. *Trauma and Recovery*. New York: Basic Books, 1991.

Hosseini, Khaled. *A Thousand Splendid Suns*. New York: Riverhead, 2007.

Kasl, Charlotte. *Women, Sex, and Addiction: A Search for Love and Power*. New York: Ticknor and Fields, 1989.

Maltz, Wendy. *The Sexual Healing Journey: A Guide for Survivors of Sexual Abuse*. Rev. ed. New York: HarperCollins, 1992.

Maltz, Wendy, and Larry Maltz. *The Porn Trap: The Essential Guide to Overcoming Problems Caused by Pornography*. New York: HarperCollins, 2008.

Najavits, Lisa. *Seeking Safety: A Treatment Manual for PTSD and Substance Abuse*. New York: Guilford Press, 2001.

Walker, Alice. *Possessing the Secret of Joy*. New York: Harcourt Brace Jovanovich, 1992.

Zoldbrod, Aline. *Sex Smart: How Your Childhood Shaped Your Sexual Life and What To Do about It*. Oakland, Calif.: New Harbinger, 1998.

Growing Older—with Infinite Variety

BOOKS

Boston Women's Health Book Collective. *Our Bodies, Ourselves: Menopause*. New York: Simon and Schuster, 2006.

Chopra, Deepak. *Ageless Body, Timeless Mind: The Quantum Alternative to Growing Old.* New York: Three Rivers Press, 1998.

Daniluk, Judith C. *Women's Sexuality across the Life Span.* Binghamton, N.Y.: Guilford Press, 1998.

Ellison, Carol. *Women's Sexualities: Generations of Women Speak about Sexual Self Acceptance.* Oakland, Calif.: New Harbinger, 2000.

Gullette, Margaret M. *Declining to Decline: Cultural Combat and the Politics of Midlife.* Charlottesville, Va.: University Press of Virginia, 1997.

Kliger, Leah, and Deborah Nedelman. *Still Sexy after All These Years? The Nine Unspoken Truths about Women's Desire beyond Fifty.* New York: Perigee, 2006.

Northrup, Christiane. *The Wisdom of Menopause: Creating Physical and Emotional Health and Healing during the Change.* Rev. ed. New York: Bantam, 2006.

DVDs

Ashby, Hal, director. *Harold and Maude.* 1971. DVD. Hollywood: Paramount, 2000.

The Science of Feeling Good—What the Researchers Say

BOOKS

Davis, Katherine Bement. *Factors in the Sex Lives of Twenty-two Hundred Women.* New York: Harper & Brothers, 1929.

Eriksen, Julia A. *Kiss and Tell: Surveying Sex in the Twentieth Century.* Cambridge, Mass.: Harvard University Press, 1999.

Fisher, Helen. *Why We Love: The Nature and Chemistry of Romantic Love.* New York: Henry Holt, 2004.

Freud, Sigmund. *"Three Contributions to the Theory of Sex."* In *The Basic Writings of Sigmund Freud.* Edited and translated by A. A. Brill. New York: Random House, 1938.

Hite, Shere. *The Hite Report: A Nationwide Study of Female Sexuality.* New York: Macmillan, 1976.

Jung, Carl G. *The Archetypes and the Collective Unconscious.* Translated by R. F. C. Hall. New York: Pantheon Books, 1959.

Kinsey, Alfred C., Wardell B. Pomeroy, and Clyde E. Martin. *Sexual Behavior in the Human Male.* Philadelphia: W. B. Saunders, 1948.

Kinsey, Alfred C., Wardell B. Pomeroy, Clyde E. Martin, and Paul H. Gebhard. *Sexual Behavior in the Human Female.* Philadelphia: W. B. Saunders, 1953.

Kleinplatz, Peggy J., ed. *New Directions in Sex Therapy: Innovations and Alternatives.* Philadelphia: Brunner-Routledge, 2001.

Kleinplatz, Peggy, and Charles Moser, eds. *Sadomasochism: Powerful Pleasures.* Binghamton, N.Y.: Harrington Park Press, 2006.

Komisaruk, Barry, Carlos Beyer, and Beverly Whipple. *The Science of Orgasm.* Baltimore: Johns Hopkins University Press, 2006.

Suggested Readings (and Viewings)

Laumann, Edward O., John H. Gagnon, Robert T. Michael, and Stuart Michaels. *The Social Organization of Sexuality: Sexual Practices in the United States.* Chicago: University of Chicago Press, 1994.

Masters, William H., and Virginia E. Johnson. *Human Sexual Response.* Boston: Little, Brown, 1966.

Ogden, Gina. "Sexuality and Spirituality in Women's Relationships: Preliminary Results of an Exploratory Survey." Working Paper 405. Wellesley, Mass.: Wellesley College Center for Research on Women, 2002.

Reich, Wilhelm. *The Function of the Orgasm.* New York: Orgone Institute Press, 1942. Reprint, translated by Vincent R. Carfagno. New York: Farrar, Straus and Giroux, 1973.

Tiefer, Leonore, and Ellyn Kaschak, eds. *A New View of Women's Sexual Problems.* Binghamton, N.Y.: Haworth Press, 2001.

Exploring the Medicine Wheel

BOOKS

Bopp, Judie. *The Sacred Tree: Reflections on Native American Spirituality.* Twin Lakes, Wis.: Lotus Press, 1984.

Lardner, Lore, and Lama Zopa Rinpoche. *The Wheel of Great Compassion: The Practice of the Prayer Wheel in Tibetan Buddhism.* Somerville, Mass.: Wisdom Publications, 2001.

Villoldo, Alberto. *The Four Insights: Wisdom, Power, and Grace of the Earthkeepers.* Carlsbad, Calif.: Hay House, 2007.

RESOURCES

On the Internet

I INVITE YOU TO VISIT MY WEBSITE: www.GinaOgden.com. Here, you'll find information and links to other websites of interest. You'll also find a downloadable ISIS survey questionnaire, additional ISIS facts, and articles about women's sexual relationships. There's also my ongoing calendar for presentations and workshops, and you can communicate directly with me through my website, so please check it out!

A special note about ISIS Connection groups. Healers around the country are offering group workshops and trainings to help you put the holistic concepts in this book into practice in your own life. My website offers information on where to locate these groups, and how you might start your own group.

Below (in alphabetical order) are other websites with information that can help you expand your thinking about sexual desire and connect you with people who are exploring similar paths. All of these organizations provide positive, culturally sensitive, pro-choice information.

- The Alexander Foundation for Women's Health. www.afwh.org
- The Bisexual Resource Center. www.biresource.org.
- College Sex Talk. www.collegesextalk.com.
- Dr. Christiane Northrup. www.DrNorthrup.com.
- Go Ask Alice! www.goaskalice.columbia.edu.
- The Intersex Society of North America. www.isna.org
- Loving More—for Polyamorous Relationships. www.lovemore.com
- The National Gay and Lesbian Task Force. www.thetaskforce.org.
- The National Women's Health Network. www.womenshealthnetwork.org
- The New View of Women's Sexuality. www.fsd-alert.org.
- Our Bodies, Ourselves. www.ourbodiesourselves.org.
- Planned Parenthood Federation of America. www.ppfa.org.
- The Sexual Health Network. www.sexualhealth.com.
- The Sexuality Information and Education Council of the United States. www.siecus.org.
- Stop It Now! www.stopitnow.org.
- Tantra.com. www.tantra.com
- The Women's Sexual Health Foundation. www.twshf.org.

Online Sexuality Boutiques

You can find thousands of sites that sell sex products, but I strongly recommend boutiques that are designed especially for women. Their websites are an education in themselves—and if you go to their physical stores, you'll find discreet, delightful environments and helpful staffs. You can purchase books and DVDs along with vibrators and other goodies for enhancing your sexual desire and pleasure. Many of these boutiques offer workshops and other educational opportunities.

- Eve's Garden in New York City. www.evesgarden.com.
- Good Vibrations in San Francisco. www.goodvibes.com.
- Toys in Babeland in New York and Seattle. www.toysinbabeland.com.
- Early to Bed in Chicago. www.early2bed.com.

Finding a Professional Sexuality Counselor

The American Association of Sexuality Educators, Counselors, and Therapists (AASECT) is an interdisciplinary organization that supervises and certifies sexuality professionals. Its members include physicians, nurses, social workers, psychologists, marriage and family therapists, clergy, lawyers, sociologists, family planning specialists, and researchers. The website provides a database of board-certified sexuality educators, counselors, and therapists all over the globe. www.aasect.org.

Finding Ongoing Sexuality Education

Several sexuality organizations offer conferences that focus on research, training, and networking with other sexuality professionals. Three of the major organizations that open their conferences to both professionals and nonprofessionals are:

- The American Association of Sexuality Educators, Counselors, and Therapists (AASECT). www.aasect.org.
- The Society for the Scientific Study of Sexuality (SSSS). www.sexscience.org.
- The International Society for the Study of Women's Sexual Health (ISSWSH). www.isswsh.org.

If you're interested in more formal study, there are a number of undergraduate and graduate programs that focus on the interdisciplinary field of human sexuality. You can find a comprehensive list on the SSSS website: www.sexscience.org.

Hotlines and Counseling

Some national hotline numbers and other sources of counseling help are listed below. For a hotline in your area, consult your local phone directory. If you are in an emergency, dial 911. If you are not in an emergency situation, take some time to check out the websites sponsored by the following resource organizations, which offer a wealth of information.

Resources

Al-Anon and Alateen (for people in relationship with substance abusers). www.alanon-alateen.org. 1-888-435-2666.

Alcoholics Anonymous (AA). www.aa.org. For a local phone number, call 411 and ask directory assistance.

Centers for Disease Control (for information about HIV/AIDS and other sexually transmitted infections). www.cdc.gov. 1-800-311-3435.

Gay, Lesbian, Transgender National Help Center. www.glnh.org. 1-888-THE-GLNH (1-888-843-4564).

National Child Abuse Hotline. www.childhelpusa.org. 1-800-4-ACHILD.

APPRECIATIONS

First and most profound gratitude goes to the 3,810 respondents of the ISIS survey, and to the hundreds of women who have participated in ISIS circles and workshops. You know who you are. This book would not exist without your stories and your courage to tell them.

Deep appreciation to my editor, Eden Steinberg, and to the entire "ISIS team" at Shambhala Publications: Laura Deily, Megan Fischer, Ben Gleason, Jonathan Green, Peter Turner, Steven Pomije, and Julie Saidenberg. You are a joy to work with.

To the women and men who have helped move ISIS consciousness in the world through sharing their wisdom, sponsoring gatherings, co-leading groups with me, inviting me to speak, publishing my work, filming me, and getting me streaming on the Web, I am grateful to Susan Bennett, Prue Berry, Stephen Braveman, Lucy Brown, Sandy Caron, Rebecca Chalker, Maril Crabtree, Cali Crowley, Jane Downing, Jean Fain, Sallie Foley, Robert Francoeur, Robert Friar, Francesca Gentile, Edith Griffin, Beth Grossman, Jennifer Gunsaullus, Judy Hancock, Judie Harvey, Suzie Heumann, Mary Hunt, Karen Hicks, Amy Joseph, Sue Katz, Carolyn Kepes, Monika Kolodziej, Wendy Maltz, Linda Marks, Tara McAvoy, John Mehr, Jaya Deb Morrissey, Emiko Omori, Rhea Orion, Annette Owens, Judy Peres, Evelyn Resh, Suzann Robins, Holly Rossi, Lou Paget, Amalya Peck, Linda Savage, Lisa Schwartz, Wendy Slick, Cynthia Snyder, Laura Stepp, Wendy Strgar, Kenneth Ray Stubbs, Michele Sugg, Mitchell Tepper, Leonore Tiefer, Barbara Thomas, Raymond Torrenti, Marilyn Volker, Dell Williams, Doug Wilson, and Ronnie Wilson (no relation).

For guidance, information, support, patience, blessing, music, and belly laughs just exactly when I needed them most, I blow special kisses to the family, friends, and colleagues who have hung in with me while I was immersed in this book—Prue Berry, Mary Bewig, Sandy Bierig, Patti Britton, Shawna Carol, Maureen Chase, Tanya Childs, Peggy Clark, Jane Claypool, Ani Colt, Maril Crabtree, Joy Davidson, Carol Ellison, Ruth Fishel, Araya Fast, Elaine Freeman, Sabine Grantke-Taft, Ruth Hannon, Karen Hicks, Jane Wegscheider Hyman, Ginny LaCrow, Loraine Hutchins, Edward Lavalle, Tara McAvoy, Ruth McConnell, Char Morrow, Alexandra Myles, Judith Nies, Nancy Nixon, Joan Duncan Oliver, Cintra Reeve, Rosemary Rossi, Cathy Saunders, Philip Saunders, Wendy Saunders, Joy Seidler, Pepita Seth, Wendy Slick, Pati Stillwater, Anne Stone, Beverly Whipple, and Judith Zaruches. And to the beloved ones who left this earth while I was writing this book: Kaye Andres, Jack Lavalle, Deborah Rose, Anne Smith, Sarah Wernick, Anne Zevin—your wit and wisdom continue to shine.

To the ISIS clinical supervision group that has met over the past year, gratitude for helping to shape the tone and direction of this book: Denise Benoit, Jo Chaffee, Sophie Glickson, Michaela Kirby, Patricia Moore, and Susan Zeichner.

Appreciations

For forums in which to present the ISIS findings and receive feedback from a wide range of professionals and nonprofessionals I thank the American Association of Sex Educators, Counselors and Therapists; the American Psychological Association; the American Public Health Association; the Association for Women in Psychology; Brigham and Women's Hospital; the Boston Area Sexuality and Spirituality Network; Canyon Ranch; Esalen Institute; the Fenway Institute; the Gerontological Society of America; Harvard Divinity School's Center for the Study of World Religions; the International Association for the Study of Dreams; the International Society for the Study of Women's Sexual Health; the Institute for Twenty-first Century Relationships; Kripalu Center for Yoga and Health; Lesley University; the National Organization for Women; the National Women's Health Network; the New View Campaign; the New York Open Center; Planned Parenthood Federation of America; the Providence Healing Center; the Radcliffe Institute; the Psychotherapy Networker; Simmons College; Rowe Conference Center; the Society for the Scientific Study of Sexuality; the Theological Opportunities Program; the Wellesley Centers for Research on Women; and the Women's Well.

For tech support that goes way beyond computer savvy, PowerPoint wizardry, or webmastery and straight to my heart—Trish Blain, Addie Escarcida, Michaela Kirby, Megan Nunnery, Bob Park, Robin Park, and Ricky Carter: you are the *best*.

To three visionaries whose brilliance and whose work has inspired me for years: Riane Eisler for the partnership wisdom that informs so much of this book, Christiane Northrup for the optimism and healing you radiate to so many women, and Judy Norsigian for teaching two generations of us how to listen to our bodies ourselves. Thank you for your contributions to this world and for your support and mentorship.

My enduring gratitude to the healers, teachers, and ceremonialists who have nurtured my body, mind, heart, and spirit in more dimensions than I thought possible: Carol Caton, Emilie Conrad, Jim Crabtree, Maribeth Kaptchuk, Lydia Knudson, Oscar Miro-Quesada, Nina Murphy, Ilene Myers, and Reva Seybolt.

And especially to Jo Chaffee, for twenty-seven years my partner, friend, and sister-researcher—you light up this book and my life.

INDEX

Index

Index

Index

Index

Index

ABOUT THE AUTHOR

DR. GINA OGDEN has had a distinguished career as a marriage and family therapist, sex therapist, teacher, researcher, and author. She has written seven books including *The Heart and Soul of Sex* and *Women Who Love Sex*. Dr. Ogden has been a featured guest on numerous radio and television programs, including *Oprah*. She lives in Cambridge, Massachusetts. For more information, visit www.GinaOgden.com.